BREATHE, SLEEP, LIVE, SMILE

INTEGRATIVE TREATMENTS FOR TMJ,
SLEEP APNEA, AND ORTHODONTICS

BREATHE,
SLEEP,
LIVE,
SMILE

DR. LYNN LIPSKIS & DR. EDMUND LIPSKIS

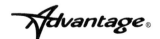

Published by Advantage, Charleston, South Carolina.
Member of Advantage Media Group.

ADVANTAGE is a registered trademark, and the Advantage colophon is a trademark of Advantage Media Group, Inc.

Printed in the United States of America.

10 9 8 7 6 5 4 3 2 1

ISBN: 978-1-59932-920-8
LCCN: 2019934488

Book design by Carly Blake.

This publication is designed to provide accurate and authoritative information in regard to the subject matter covered. It is sold with the understanding that the publisher is not engaged in rendering legal, accounting, or other professional services. If legal advice or other expert assistance is required, the services of a competent professional person should be sought.

Advantage Media Group is proud to be a part of the Tree Neutral® program. Tree Neutral offsets the number of trees consumed in the production and printing of this book by taking proactive steps such as planting trees in direct proportion to the number of trees used to print books. To learn more about Tree Neutral, please visit **www.treeneutral.com**.

Advantage Media Group is a publisher of business, self-improvement, and professional development books and online learning. We help entrepreneurs, business leaders, and professionals share their Stories, Passion, and Knowledge to help others Learn & Grow. Do you have a manuscript or book idea that you would like us to consider for publishing? Please visit **advantagefamily.com** or call **1.866.775.1696**.

This book is dedicated to all of the wonderful people who have helped us develop these protocols: our mentors, our patients, our staff, and our family.

To Ed, my wonderful, brilliant husband who has worked tirelessly to process all that he has learned into a logical sequence of treatment.

To Lynn, my amazing wife, who has been the driving force in our quest to help our patients. Thanks for always having my back.

Thank you to our parents—Louis and Irene Orlowski, and Antanas and Alina Lipskis—who started us on life's journey in the right direction. They raised us to "do it right." It is that mantra that has brought us to this point in our lives.

And last but not least, thanks to our three wonderful daughters (Kristina, Laura, and Dana) who at times were "test subjects" even though they did not know it. They have been supportive of our quest and hopefully understand how it has benefited them.

TABLE OF CONTENTS

ACKNOWLEDGMENTS

Thank you to Dr. Steven Olmos, who took all of our extensive, yet scattered knowledge, and helped us organize it into a comprehensive protocol. We appreciate your friendship.

Thank you to Dr. Romano, Dr. Klauer, Dr. Cantieri, Dr. Wells, Dr. Geivelis, Dr. Boyd, Dr. Desai, Dr. Shrivastava, Dr. Hestrup, Dr. Loghmanee, Dr. Mahony, and Dr. Marquina for all the information and support you have given us throughout the years.

Thank you to Dr. Marcus and Dr. Billings for your unfailing friendship throughout the years and being a great sounding board for ideas.

A big shout out to our associate dentists—Dr. Dana and Dr. Lisa—who support our quest and realize how important it is for their patients' health. You guys rock!

Thank you to our office staff who stuck with us throughout all the "change" that needed to occur in our thinking and practice protocols to create a system that works. And thank you for your patience to this day as we continue our quest for more information to improve what we do.

Thank you to all the wonderful people who have entrusted us with their health care and continue to refer friends and family because they believe in what we do.

FOREWORD

DEEPAK SHRIVASTAVA,
MD, FAASM, FCCP, FACP

M any years ago, on a beautiful summer morning in Scottsdale, Arizona, just before starting a dental sleep medicine course, I had the pleasure of meeting a wonderful couple—Drs. Edmund and Lynn Lipskis. We met in a hurry but later that evening, we sat at the same dinner table and got to know one another. I discovered then that this couple is different, mature, and very knowledgeable. We quickly developed mutual respect and understanding. This was the beginning of a long journey and an academic pursuit that still continues.

Recently when Drs. Edmund and Lynn Lipskis asked me to write a foreword for their new book *Breathe, Sleep, Live, Smile: Integrative Treatments for TMJ, Sleep Apnea, and Orthodontics*, I felt deeply honored. Knowing their background preparation of over four decades and their well-known mentors, and seeing endorsements of their competence by multiple boards, I instantly knew that their book was going to be a novel testament in the field of TMD, sleep apnea, chronic pain, and other ailments related to the human airway.

Both chronic craniofacial pain and sleep disordered breathing are underestimated in current epidemiologic studies. These disorders span from infancy to old age. In the practice of sleep medicine, there are numerous questions and very few answers. Drs. Lipskis entered a difficult time in their academic careers when Lynn suffered with severe TMD. Ed decided to take all his knowledge and expertise and began to work with Lynn, applying all of it to orthodontics in new ways. By this time, Edmund had met his TMD mentor, Dr. Steven Olmos.

The first sign of wisdom is to be able to apply learned knowledge and education to improve human health in both conventional and novel ways. Edmund's reward came in the form of resolution of Lynn's chronic TMJ pain problems. There was proof that this technique works.

Edmund and Lynn both expanded on their experience and continued to study their patients to fine-tune their technique. They put their treatment method to the ultimate test and successfully treated their three daughters who had the same problem that Lynn had suffered with. Edmund wrote, "the resulting beautiful smiles were the reward, but better sleep and improved airways was an incredible bonus."

They recognized the fact that obstructed airway in sleep disordered breathing begins in the very early years of life. They recognized the implications of tongue-tie and difficulty with breast-feeding as the infant is unable to get their tongue under the mother's nipple. Breast-feeding over the months shapes the development of infant's airway and prevents sleep-disordered breathing in the future. An early intervention is invaluable in avoiding long-term damage to organ systems including brain, heart, metabolic system and neurocognitive problems.

Such approach requires a thorough understanding of the relationship between the human anatomy and physiology—the interaction between the structure and function of human organ systems. In this book, Lynn and Ed provide excellent education to readers by simplifying complex concepts. They empower the reader to become part of a knowledgeable team so that the reader can participate in their own care. Chapter after chapter, the authors continue to describe the inseparable relationship between TMJ, sleep apnea, and chronic pain. It becomes very clear that a complete understanding of all three components is really important for the assessment and successful treatment of these disorders.

One of the worse miseries of human life is to give up hope. For the people suffering with chronic pain and sleep disordered breathing, the hope lies in finding a knowledgeable provider who understands the finer shades and nuances of airway development and the intricate relationship between poor sleep quality and worsening pain. The authors have spread their wealth of knowledge and experience by educating hundreds of dental healthcare providers over the years.

Overall, this is a long-awaited and thought-provoking book that fulfills the gap in applied knowledge; thinking through the human physiology and making sense out of the science. This explores the mostly blurred lines between the normal and the abnormal. It reflects the quest to find the truth; for once the truth is discovered, the cure isn't much farther!

Deepak Shrivastava, MD, FAASM, FCCP, FACP

Professor of Sleep Medicine, Pulmonary and Critical Care,
UC Davis School of Medicine, Sacramento California
Senior faculty, University of California Davis ACGME
accredited Sleep Fellowship program
Director, Sleep Diagnostics Center, SJGH, Stockton California

t is my sincere pleasure and honor to have been asked to write this for my good friends and colleagues, Drs. Lynn and Ed Lipskis. They are a powerful combination and a vital resource for the city of Chicago.

They are unique in their quest and thirst for knowledge. I know that almost every weekend they're attending a continued education course, and every waking moment that they're not helping people is spent reading. I am awed by their perseverance.

This drive for knowledge is only surpassed by their true caring for all people who struggle with chronic pain and breathing disorders. They exemplify the title "Doctor," and give back to their communities with their professional skills in education, law, and dentistry. They demonstrated their compassion and caring by raising three wonderful and talented women—defining what we should all strive to be as parents. I feel gifted by their presence.

I write this describing "them" as they share a common path, however, they are two different people with unique skills. Lynn is driven to free people from the chronic pain she has experienced in her life. I can relate to that mission. She looks for the origin of pain, understanding that there will be a cascade of relief for symptoms. Ed has special skills in understanding how to transform—through non-surgical, orthopedic/orthodontic therapy—the distortions of the skull that are the result of functional problems (functional problems being the essential functions of life, such as breathing). Proper breathing is through the nose, not the mouth.

This book reviews the path they took to gain the abilities to help so many people. They give scientific reasons and empathize them with examples of real people they have helped. They cover a good amount of material and make it easy to read and assimilate.

I am very proud of Lynn and Ed and their efforts in writing this book that will help so many people.

Sincerely,

Steven R. Olmos

DABCP, DABCDSM, DAIPM, DABDSM,

FAAOP, FAACP, FICCMO, FADI, FIAO

Founder, TMJ & Sleep Therapy Centres International

INTRODUCTION
A Journey For Answers

How many people can say every day that they have changed someone else's life? That's the joy and passion that drives us daily in our work. What began as a personal "mini" crusade, we now recognize as a worldwide epidemic. Unfortunately, this epidemic has not been recognized by most health care providers.

More than 11 percent of Americans suffer one or more symptoms of chronic craniofacial pain.[1] Over twenty-five million Americans have sleep apnea, and the numbers for diabetes and other metabolic disorders are skyrocketing![2]

Children are really having issues with sleep apnea, and its impact has increased on adolescents in the past thirty years. Dr. Stephen Sheldon of Lourie Children's Hospital in Chicago says 20 to 25 percent

---

1   Lecia Bushak, "The Stress of Severe Pain: 11% of Americans Suffer From Chronic Pain, NIH States," Medical Daily, August 11, 2015, https://www.medicaldaily.com/stress-severe-pain-11-americans-suffer-chronic-pain-nih-states-347292.

2   "Rising prevalence of sleep apnea in U.S. threatens public health," American Academy of Sleep Medicine, September 29, 2014, https://aasm.org/rising-prevalence-of-sleep-apnea-in-u-s-threatens-public-health.

of ADHD diagnosed children have sleep apnea as the causative factor.[3]

We have been in private practice for more than thirty-seven years as of this writing (2018), and from 1982 to 1993, we were associate professors in the Department of Pediatric Dentistry at Loyola University of Chicago. Helping people who have been to numerous providers and received numerous treatments—none of which really resolved their problems—brings enormous satisfaction to both of us. Every day, we get to "do the impossible" as one patient described during our treatment for her.

Of course, it helps to know what it's like to actually be that patient suffering from a mysterious disorder that no provider has answers for. We also understand the joy that accompanies recovering from the constant pain and confusion, and what it's like to have the restoration of hope.

What people do not realize is that answers are not one size fits all when you are dealing with humans who are not healthy. And the patient is the most important team member on their health recovery team.

Beginning in the early 1980s, Lynn suffered from a disorder of the temporomandibular joints (TMJ)—the joint in the jaw that causes so many people pain and presents a wide variety of symptoms. As a teen, she had already undergone conventional orthodontics: extractions, retraction (wearing head gear), tooth reshaping, and braces. As a young adult, she often suffered from migraines and pain in her neck and back—areas of the body that, at the time, didn't seem to point to her jaws as the culprit. She had to cope, and often blamed the aches and pains on her work as a dentist, especially all the "hunching over." At the time, no one in conventional health care really knew how to identify or address Lynn's problems—the TMJ was a mystery that no one really

---

3   "Dr. Stephen Sheldon Explains the Importance of Sleep Evaluations in Children," American Academy of Physiological Medicine & Dentistry, May 8, 2013, video, 6:58, https://youtu.be/wz5kDoyPRe4.

understood at the time. Physicians (even orthopedists) weren't taught about the TM joint and didn't want to "own" the problems associated with jaw joints. Dentists weren't trained to diagnose or treat it either. So, the TMJ was an "orphan" part of the body, of sorts, that no one really wanted to take responsibility for. This unfortunate situation continues to this day.

Together, we embarked upon a journey to try to figure out a solution for Lynn's chronic pain problems. Finally, while attending an orthodontic seminar featuring the speaker John Witzig, DDS (considered by many to be the father of functional orthodontics in the United States), Lynn realized that she shared symptoms with a patient he was talking about. On our drive home from Minneapolis, Lynn made the decision to undergo orthodontics for the second time. It was 1985 and Ed would be attempting to undo some of the retraction and damage done by her adolescent treatment.

At the present time, Ed's practice focuses on airway-directed orthodontics and evaluating patients from a skeletal, airway, and balance standpoint. From a health standpoint, straightening the teeth often seems like a secondary priority. This is because when the face is made more symmetric and in balance, the smile turns out to be even more amazing than previously thought possible. So, medical/structural issues are addressed first, because the deficient or aberrant facial development seen today leads to those types of issues. Thirty years ago, it was a challenge and much of the necessary research and technology had not been completed. Using his expertise and a lot of thought, Ed was able to figure out a way to develop Lynn's deficient midface (face, cheekbones, nose, and mouth) forward so that her lower jaw was no longer being held back, which was a significant factor in the symptoms she was experiencing.

The quest to further our knowledge continued in 2000, when

we began seeking out and consulting with the experts in the field to resolve problems we were seeing with patients. Lynn was looking for specific answers to the TMJ puzzle, and Ed was taking what was already known in orthodontics and the TMJ field and applying it to orthodontics in new ways.

In 2001, when we attended a seminar with orthodontist Derek Mahony of Australia, several attendees mentioned Steven Olmos, DDS. They mentioned that Dr. Olmos had spent several years developing a new protocol, which sounded exactly like what we were looking for to resolve craniofacial pain in patients we were seeing.

Shortly after that, we met Dr. Olmos when he was teaching a course in Chicago, and what he presented made a lot of sense. He had been able to take the varied fields of knowledge and condense them into a logical protocol. Lynn decided to try Dr. Olmos's protocol for craniofacial pain. She had an appliance made to the specifications Olmos taught, including applying the technique for determining the best jaw position, and wore it as prescribed. She soon began noticing less discomfort while working.

Soon after, a family emergency required her to travel to Connecticut from Chicago, alone. At that time, she was typically unable to ride in a car more than a couple of hours without experiencing severe back pain. After starting treatment with the appliance she'd made for herself, she wore it while driving sixteen hours straight from Chicago to Connecticut to be by her mother's side. Later, she realized that she had not experienced pain during the entire drive.

Two weeks later, after she had returned home and was raking leaves, she realized that she was able to rake for hours without any pain. That was the "aha" moment that made her question: could a simple oral orthotic (made correctly) change posture and body mechanics, and eliminate pain and inflammation so significantly?

Up to that point, we had limited our involvement in treating TMJ, but after Lynn's experience, it was an easy decision to follow Dr. Olmos's protocol. This protocol has consistently produced predictable results. And the results are truly profound, as you'll see in some of the case studies presented in the chapters ahead.

By 2010, Lynn had completely evolved from general dentistry and limited her practice to treating temporomandibular joint disorders; undiagnosed, chronic pain; and sleep apnea, as these conditions are inexorably linked.

While Lynn's practice was evolving, Ed was also changing his practice to concentrate on orthodontics for children and adults. Over time, he found that patients still had posture, pain, and breathing issues that the traditional orthodontics he'd been trained in couldn't seem to resolve. Convinced that there had to be better treatment options, he continued to look for answers to deliver what his patients clearly needed.

The evolution of Ed's practice truly was a labor of love. We have three daughters who, as young children, were in serious need of orthodontic care. Since Lynn had dealt with so many of her own problems, we were determined to find a solution for our daughters that would not involve extracting permanent teeth, a type of treatment that is still considered the standard of care and a normal part of orthodontics. That didn't make sense to us. So, necessity definitely became the mother of invention. Ed worked out strategies to maximize the growth of their jaws, grow new bone structure, and was able to avoid extracting any teeth on our girls, despite significant dental crowding. The resulting beautiful smiles were the reward, but better sleep and improved airways were an incredible bonus.

Ed has spent thirty years developing what today is a unique system of facial orthopedics that moves teeth and develops deficient dentofacial-skeletal features, using what looks like conventional orthodontics, but which functions very differently.

Today, he teaches his system to other dentists and orthodontists around the world, some that travel from great distances for this unique program. It also provides hands-on training with patients.

The purpose of this book is to share with patients and consumers a new practice model designed to get people healthier. The more patients know, the more they will ask their providers for the treatments that are integrated with other types of care to treat the whole patient. It is a shift in the usual medical mind set, providing *health* care, not care for disease symptoms. The patient experiences described in this book are real. We have altered the identities to ensure their privacy.

At the Centre for Integrative Orthodontics, we believe healthy smiles are beautiful smiles.

Who doesn't want to be happier, healthier, better looking, stronger, sleep better, and feel rested? That's the goal of these treatments, and the goal of us sharing the information found in the pages ahead. It's a win across the board for both patients and providers.

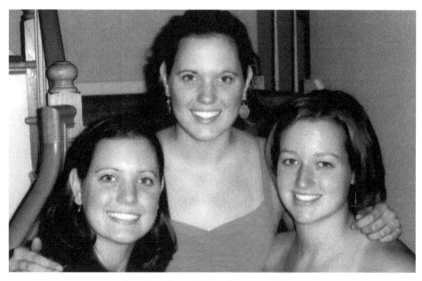

Our daughters: Kristina, Laura, and Dana

CHAPTER 1

The Need to Breathe

I f you're driving down a highway and accidentally get off at the wrong exit ramp, and then realize what you've done when you're at the bottom of the ramp, it's easy to correct your mistake. You simply cross over to the on-ramp, zip back onto the highway, and get back on your way. But, if you don't recognize the mistake immediately, you may find yourself miles away, in the middle of the woods somewhere, with no convenient ramp for reentering the highway you mistakenly left. If you keep going forward, blissfully ignorant, you end up going farther in the wrong direction. And the farther you go, the longer the trip and the more difficult it is to get back on the correct highway.

That illustrates one of the points of our little "crusade." We strive to inform parents of the needs of their children so that we can get them back on the "road to health" as quickly and simply as possible. Where mainstream orthodontists say they want to first see children at age seven, we want to see them as newborns for tongue tie evaluation and possible correction, and as two- to five-year-olds to correct growth issues, and to change incorrect function to ideal function.

For people who are dealing with problems such as TMJ, facial development issues, crooked teeth, and sleep apnea, waiting is not a good idea. Oftentimes TMJ and sleep apnea are not addressed until adulthood. But by evaluating kids at a very early age for the problems that can ultimately lead to TMJ and sleep apnea, we can keep them "on the right track" and help them avoid some of the issues that adults face. If an evaluation determines that a child is not on the right track, then it's easier to get them back on that track if intervention is done as soon as possible. The correction at a young age is much smaller and much easier to make. The result is also much more stable. Once a correction is made with function normalized, nature takes over and children will continue to develop into healthy individuals who are less likely to need braces or treatment for TMJ/sleep apnea later in life. They will have been set back on the correct road to a healthy life.

Humans Need Air/Oxygen

The importance of breathing to maintain life is second to none. Humans can go forty days without food, and eight days without water—but only minutes without air. Oxygen is the most important nutrient for the human body. Without proper breathing during sleep, the oxygen levels needed by the body cannot be maintained, leading to various health issues. That includes physical and psychological conditions, which can be life-threatening, along with cognitive issues.

That's why the brain's highest priority is maintaining a flow of oxygen into the body. It does this by pacing breathing (fast versus slow) and by repositioning the head and neck when needed to maintain an open airway.

Breathing is so important that we are all equipped with two intake sources—the nose and the mouth. The primary and healthiest intake is through the nose, which, among other advantages, cleans, warms, moistens, and reduces the velocity of air before it hits the lungs. The mouth is a secondary or "backup" intake. Since the air that enters the lungs through the mouth is dry, dirty, cold, and moving at an irritatingly high velocity, it's important to regularly breathe through the nose to maintain a strong immune system and overall health.

If the airway is compromised or obstructed for some reason, the brain puts such a high priority on addressing the problem that it will actually change the way a person stands just to find the best position to open their airway—even to the point of straining, or even causing damage to, other areas of the body. This may lead to a point where pain from these strained or injured body parts occurs. This happens because changing the posture of the head and neck to open the throat (the oropharyngeal airway) is more important to the brain than straining or even causing some injury to the body parts involved in maintaining the postural changes.

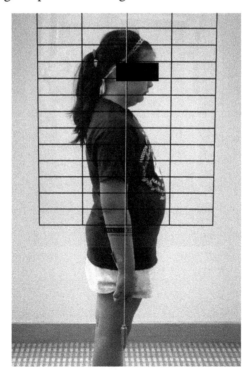

These postural changes are essentially the same concept used in cardiopulmonary resuscitation (CPR), where the rescuer elevates the chin to open the airway enough to allow the resuscitator to breathe air into the victim.

We are currently implementing breathing analysis and Buteyko breathing instructions into our protocols to help people learn to breathe through their nose. We cannot overstate the importance of using your nose to provide clean, warm, and healthy air, and to control loss of carbon dioxide to help maintain your health.

In our office, we utilize the latest technology to get the most accurate diagnostic information possible. During our evaluation of patients, we use state-of-the-art, three-dimensional cone beam imaging. It's not uncommon to find that their airway is nearly fully obstructed, even when they are awake and upright—imagine what happens to their airway and breathing when they are unconscious and lying on their back! That's when sleep apnea—a form of sleep-disordered breathing caused by an obstructed airway, occurs.

With obstructive sleep apnea (OSA), a blocked airway causes the brain to arouse from a deep, restful sleep to open the airway so the sleeper can breathe. This arousal does not usually result in full wakefulness, but represents a change in the state of sleep. The change results in fragmented, lighter stages of sleep and a loss of the advantages of the uninterrupted, deep, restful, and recuperative sleep. Our patients often are not aware that they are not sleeping soundly, as they do not become fully conscious.

Complete airway blockage occurs at night when a person lies down to sleep and their muscles relax to the point of collapsing in on some part of their airway. At that point, the brain takes emergency action. Its primary role is to keep the body alive, so it will arouse the person to a lighter level of sleep, but it usually does not fully wake them. That arousal action changes the muscle tone in the airway, causing the muscles to increase tone, and to open the airway, allowing the sleeper to breathe again. This cycle often repeats itself many times each night. The person falls back to sleep for a little bit and breathes adequately, then the muscles surrounding the airway begin to relax as deeper sleep sets in. The airway collapses again, initiating the brain's survival response, arousing the person to a lighter stage of sleep and opening the airway. Strangely, the person is not aware that this is happening because they are "asleep." The difficulty is that their sleep is disturbed and that can lead to anxiety, depression, or other medical conditions such as diabetes and hypertension.[4]

The airway collapse can occur in different ways. It can be the muscles relaxing and causing an actual narrowing of the throat portion of the airway, or it can be the tongue falling back into the throat and blocking it, or it can even be nasal passages that become congested and closed. Whatever the cause, the result is the same: the airway gets blocked. Unblocking it can only be accomplished by going from deeper, more restful, recuperative stages of sleep into shallower sleep that is not as beneficial.

Sleep is essential—humans must sleep for the body to be restored and for their brain to function normally.

Currently, it is taught that there are five levels of consciousness/ sleep: Stage 0 (awake); Stage 1 (light sleep); Stage 2 (you are asleep fully); Stage 3 (deep recuperative sleep); REM (Rapid Eye Movement) sleep. In stage 1 and 2, the body begins to relax and fall asleep. Stage 3 sleep is deeper than the first two and is the stage of sleep when the body physically repairs or recuperates. It is the stage in which growth mainly occurs in children. REM sleep is important for cognitive devel-

---

4   Schimita Pamidi, Renee Aronson, and Esra Tasal, "Obstructive Sleep Apnea: Role in the Risk and Severity of Diabetes," *Best Practice & Research: Clinical Endocrinology & Metabolism* 24, no. 5 (October 2010): 703–715, https://doi.org/10.1016/j.beem.2010.08.009.

opment and learning. During REM sleep, nearly all the voluntary muscles in the body completely relax, unlike the involuntary muscles like the heart, which keeps beating, and the diaphragm, which keeps you breathing. Sleep that is constantly disrupted reduces the ability to maintain a deep, restorative Stage 3 sleep, let alone make it into REM sleep.

The problems of OSA are most severe when the sufferer is in REM sleep, since that's when the brain forms new neural pathways, detoxifies, and recharges. In adults, constant disruptions of REM diminish what is known as executive function—essentially, memory, impulse control, decision-making, and activity levels. In children, chronic interruptions of REM can lead to cognitive developmental issues of their brain. Since a child's brain grows at an accelerated rate during REM sleep, it is constantly being pulled out of that regenerative state, which prevents the brain from reaching its full potential. That can lead to permanent brain deficits in kids. Research from Johns Hopkins has shown that if correction is not made early enough, permanent cognitive deficits can occur.[5]

The reduced oxygen to the brain prevents neuronal pathways from being formed, and in severe cases, evidence has shown that existing neuronal pathways are destroyed. That is the really upsetting part of sleep disorders in kids—their cognitive abilities (learning, reasoning, and memory)—can be limited or lessened by sleep apnea. During a single night's sleep, it is optimal to go through four to eight sleep cycles (each cycle being sixty to ninety minutes in length). Until a person can stay asleep long enough to naturally cycle all the way through REM several times during sleep, their problems will continue—and potentially worsen.

---

5   Johns Hopkins Medical Institutions, "Childhood Sleep Apnea Linked to Brain Damage, Lower IQ," *Science Daily,* August 27, 2006, accessed at www.sciencedaily.com/releases/2006/08/060826171825.htm.

The body has the ability to compensate for pain by repositioning itself into a variety of postures, some of which can ultimately damage or strain other areas. For instance, the forward head posture (FHP) can place additional strains on muscles and joints of the neck because they are not being used in the manner they were designed for. When an area of the body is forced to function in a way it wasn't designed to function, the result can be pain or even loss of function.

The airway is no exception. When a person's breathing is more difficult because their nose is blocked, the body will compensate and possibly cause injury/symptoms. For instance, if the nasal passages become obstructed during sleep and cause the person to struggle to breathe, then their jaw will shift position in an effort to open their airway. When the jaw shifts side to side or front to back and the teeth are in contact, a person is doing what's known as "grinding" of their teeth. As their oxygen levels lower and carbon dioxide, or CO_2 builds up, then their masseter muscles (the large cheek muscles) contract, causing what's known as "clenching." While the grinding can severely damage teeth, the clenching creates a lot of stress by compressing the jaw joint.

If clenching and grinding is being caused by a closed nasal passage at the entry point (inferior nasal valve), then the problem can be reduced with nasal strips or nasal valves. Any blockage higher up may respond to nasal spray, or to a more permanent surgical procedure to open the nasal airway. These "permanent" solutions include orthodontic palatal expansion and/or surgery. It may also involve nasal surgery performed by a highly trained ENT. Sometimes the beneficial effects of treating a problem can be immediate. For instance, time-lapsed photography has actually demonstrated how certain procedures or treatments (such as nasal spray or laser therapy) can instantly cause a person to upright their "crooked" stance when their posture is the result of a breathing problem.

Problems resulting from lack of sleep

- Premature death
- Hypertension, heart disease
- Abnormal growth patterns
- Asymmetry of the face
- Cognitive deficits
- ADHD-like symptoms
- Sleep apnea
- TMJ/TMD
- Joint issues
- Sore neck or back
- Diabetes
- Weight gain, obesity
- Excessive Daytime Sleepiness
- Erectile Dysfunction

There is a connection between disrupted sleep and debilitating disease. A lot of physical issues can happen when a person is constantly being pulled out of Stage 3 sleep. Those physical problems occur largely as a result of inflammation. When the body becomes chronically inflamed, it can more easily develop problems such as weight gain (and all the issues associated with that), diabetes, cancer, and hypertension—leading to heart attack or stroke.[6]

---

6   David Gozal, Ramon Farre, and F. Javier Nieto, "Putative Links Between Sleep Apnea and Cancer," *Chest* 148, no. 5 (November 2015): 1140–1147, https://doi.org/10.1378/chest.15-0634.

TMJ or TMD?

Most people refer to problems associated with their jaw joint as TMJ. But TMJ technically refers to the actual joint in the jaw itself—the temporomandibular joint. The collection of problems associated with the TMJ are actually known as TMDs (temporomandibular disorders) or TMJD (temporomandibular joint disorders).

To avoid confusion, throughout the rest of the book, we'll refer to the disorders associated with the temporomandibular joint as TMJ, the more commonly used term.

Sympathetic Versus Parasympathetic

Just as the brain sends up an alarm when breathing is disrupted during sleep, it also sends up an alarm when there is pain or an injury somewhere in the body that the brain perceives as severe enough to cause a loss of function or is a threat to survival. That alarm, which results in significant changes in the way the body functions, is commonly known as "fight-or-flight."

Fight-or-flight is the body's automatic reaction to a real or perceived situation of danger. When the body is in fight-or-flight, it automatically starts pumping more adrenaline, cortisol, and other hormones to help the organism run away from or combat the threat.

For instance, if an injury in the knee makes it difficult to walk properly for some time, then the brain resorts to a primitive way of thinking. It perceives that pain and loss of function in the knee as true danger, to the point of lowering the body's ability to survive.

If the brain detects it has a significant injury, the only mechanism it has to protect itself is to place the body into a fight-or-flight state, what is neurologically termed a *sympathetic state*. Under normal circumstances, the fight-or-flight state is supposed to be transient—it turns on and off only as needed for relatively short emergency situations. But when the brain constantly senses a potential survival threat, fight-or-flight may become a long-term condition. It stays turned on all the time, causing the body to continuously remain in a hypervigilant, emergency state to deal with the "threats," or in this case, pain or injury. Without a conscious effort, the body will change posture or alter its development to protect the damaged site and maintain its ability to function as optimally as possible.

For example, if there is injury in the neck from damaged vertebrae but moving the neck sideways and forward a little puts those vertebrae in a protected position, then the brain will make that happen. And it makes that happen all the time without the person consciously realizing it—that's the compensatory, adaptive, or protective posture. Unfortunately, placing the body in that protective position then forces another area of the body to alter the way it functions—the opposite shoulder, for instance, may be stretched to the point of eventually causing pain. But in the sympathetic state, the brain has decided that protecting the injured area (the vertebrae) is more important to survival than the pain that the opposite shoulder is feeling. That's why correcting one area of the body can actually reduce or eliminate pain in another area—correcting the injured vertebrae is the way to eliminate the pain in the shoulder, in our example above.

When a body is in a sympathetic state, the heart rate elevates, the adrenal glands work overtime to pump out hormones to handle the crisis, the thyroid gland will kick into overdrive, digestion is interrupted—all while peripheral blood flow is reduced. All of these (and additional) activities occur because, in flight-or-flight, the body is preparing to defend itself, to survive. It's in a chronic state of emergency. Basically, physiologically, the body thinks it's constantly being chased by a tiger, even when there's no tiger on the loose.

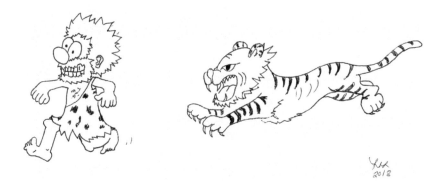

Living in a sympathetic state is hard on the body. Patients in this state are frequently misdiagnosed with conditions such as chronic fatigue syndrome or fibromyalgia.

Even sleeping becomes more of a problem, because the body never is able to enter a restful state. In time, that hyperactive, hyper-vigilant state can lead to issues such as insomnia or chronic tiredness. While sleep may come, since the brain is continually monitoring the injury, and constantly "looking for the tiger," you're more likely to wake up—over and over again.

Parasympathetic is the opposite of the sympathetic state. It's a more relaxed state, also known as "rest-and-digest." Even though this is the more "desired state," it can contribute to breathing issues. Since REM sleep is a parasympathetic state, the likelihood of the nasal passages becoming obstructed or blocked is more likely at night than at any time during the day. Even a nose that's normally not blocked can become blocked in REM sleep, especially if there's already a little bit of conges-tion. A blocked nose forces breathing through the mouth, leading to a host of negative consequences, including snoring. The alternative to mouth-breathing is an obstructive apnea event described previously as an interruption in breathing that leads to an arousal event.

Sleep Problems Also Plague Kids

Breathing disruptions are problematic enough for adults but imagine how damaging it can be to kids. Unfortunately, parents often are not aware of or overlook the sleep problems their child is having. Or, what's worse, children are misdiagnosed and placed on medication as a result of their symptoms.

Sleep problems can manifest symptoms and present as behavioral issues, such as ADHD or learning disabilities. Many kids are misdiagnosed with ADHD and are put on medications such as Adderall or Ritalin, which are stimulants.[7]

Now, ADHD is most likely a real diagnosis, but too often children do not have the condition. Rather, they have issues that are treatable without medications. When a child has sleep apnea, they're not resting well. They are constantly waking to breathe. Their brain is not getting the oxygen it needs. That can lead to physical changes to the brain—the prefrontal cortex not developing at the normal rate—which can lead to the ADHD-like symptoms.

In children suffering from disrupted sleep, the solution is to fix the sleep apnea, and it is best to address that at the earliest age possible—as soon as it is detected. That can help eliminate the chance that the child will develop a permanent brain deficit. With children, there really is a window of opportunity to make things right. Neuropathways can be developed at any point in life—that's how adults continue to learn new things. However, learning as an adult does not take place at the rapid rate that it occurs during childhood, due to

---

7   Louise M. O'Brien et al., "Neurobehavioral Correlates of Sleep-Disordered Breathing in Children," *Journal of Sleep Research* 13, no.2 (May 26, 2004): 165–172, https://doi.org/10.1111/j.1365-2869.2004.00395.x.

the accelerated rate of brain growth and neural pathway formation in young children (see chart below).

HUMAN BRAIN DEVELOPMENT
Synapse Formation Dependent on Early Experiences

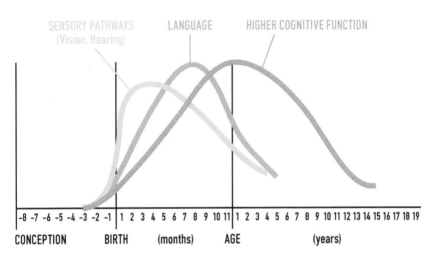

SENSORY PATHWAYS (Vision, Hearing)   LANGUAGE   HIGHER COGNITIVE FUNCTION

-8 -7 -6 -5 -4 -3 -2 -1 | 1 2 3 4 5 6 7 8 9 10 11 | 1 2 3 4 5 6 7 8 9 10 11 12 13 14 15 16 17 18 19

CONCEPTION   BIRTH   (months)   AGE   (years)

Source: Nelson (2000)

We've seen these symptoms or signs in teens who are nearing adulthood when the window of opportunity was missed. They're not unintelligent, but they struggle because of limited focus. If they do not find a subject in school interesting, then they will not learn. They may concentrate on a new piece of information that captures their attention, learn it, and even master it. But other information falls to the wayside because of the deficiency for neural pathway development in the brain—all because their sleep apnea wasn't addressed during their formative years.

The growth curve of the brain, especially for executive and cognitive functions, accelerates from birth until the age of twelve. If there's a deficiency in the neural pathway and brain growth isn't corrected during that time, then it is really too late to avoid some permanent cognitive deficits. At that point, the child has left the highway and the re-entry ramp (return to the most ideal brain development) is closed for good.

CHAPTER 2
The Changing Face of Man

t has been documented that over time, diet has led to changes in the shape of the human body. In our lifetimes, we've seen that in the chronic weight gain that plagues modern man.

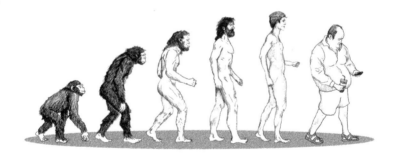

There is one area of the body that has undergone significant transformation in a short period of time, and it's affecting the health of the body as a whole. We're talking about the human face. Today's average face is much smaller than that of early humans, and this is often attributed to what is known as the Standard American Diet (SAD), which is high in processed and refined foods, fried and junk foods, fatty meat and dairy, and carbohydrates and sugar. And yes, the SAD is, indeed, very sad.[8]

There are many sources of information on this subject, beginning with Weston Price. Interestingly, over ten thousand years ago, human beings were taller than they are now and their brains were larger in size than they are today. With the advent of agriculture, everything started to change because of the introduction of grains and the availability of foods with higher carbohydrate content. These carbohydrates promote inflammation, which in and of itself also tends to inhibit growth.

Anthropologically, from preagricultural times, the human body and brain gradually continued to decline in size until the mid-1700s.[9] Then it took a turn for the worse as the British Tea Company became very efficient at providing sugar to the world from Central America and the Caribbean. With sugar becoming increasingly available, faces got even smaller and bellies got bigger.

The second negative aspect of a processed, high-carbohydrate diet is that it is soft and does not require a lot of chewing. Jaw development relies upon the stimulus of chewing harder foods at an early age.[10] Dr. German Ramirez-Yanez, a pedodontist, has written numerous articles dealing with breast feeding and early childhood diets.[11] Dr. Kevin Boyd is investigating the differences in the jaw structures from an anthropologic aspect and has coined the phrase "Craniofacial Man-

8   P. W. Lucas. "Facial Dwarfing and Dental Crowding in Relation to Diet," *International Congress Series* 1296 (June 2006): 74–82; D. Lieberman, *The Story of the Human Body: Evolution, Health and Disease* (UK: Penguin UK) (Kindle Locations 5194–5195); Lynne Oliver, "Food Timeline FAQS: Baby Food," *Food Time Library*, http://bit.ly/292HXnw.

9   John Hawks, "How has the human brain evolved over the years?" *Scientific American Mind* 24, no. 3 (July 2013).

10   Robert Corruccini, *How Anthropology Informs the Orthodontic Diagnosis of Malocclusion's Causes (Mellen Studies in Anthropology, 1)* (Lewiston: Edwin Mellen, 1999); Daniel Liebermann, *The Story of the Human Body: Evolution, Health, and Disease* (London: Penguin Books, 2014).

11   S. Kufley, J.E. Scott, and G. Ramirez-Yanez, "The Effect or Physical Consistency of the Diet on the Bone Quality," *Archives of Oral Biology* 77 (May 2017): 23–26, https://doi.org/10.1016/j.archoralbio.2017.01.015.

dibular Respiratory Morphology."[12]

We feed infants with a bottle, which creates abnormal oral muscle function, then wean them onto ground-up fruits and vegetables. From there, toddlers are given heavily processed "adult" food which does not require a lot of chewing. It is no wonder we have observed a definite trend of underdeveloped jaws and constricted nasal and oropharyngeal airways. The trend has not only continued to present day, but it is actually accelerating.

In the last fifty years, fat was condemned as the major culprit in heart disease—this has now been shown to be completely incorrect—and sugar was added to many of our foods to improve taste and texture. In response to the changing opinions, sugar is now being taken out of food and replaced with sugar substitutes. The idea was to reduce the calories that the sugar added. This is still not a workable solution. These sugar substitutes actually trick the brain into an insulin response (which is the normal response to ingesting sugar). Since no real sugar is being consumed, the insulin remains in your blood stream, causing cravings to eat even more sugar to address all of the insulin produced by the sugar substitute insulin spike. The result is high blood insulin levels, which cause people to eat sugar to meet the insulin supply—a never-ending eating cycle! The result is Type 2 Diabetes, or a less severe state of Insulin Resistance. Both conditions have been connected to weight gain and heart disease. The latest CDC statistics report that nearly one-third of Americans are diabetic or "prediabetic."[13]

---

12   K. L. Boyd,"Darwinian Dentistry Part 2: Early Childhood Nutrition, Dento-Facial Development and Chronic Disease," *J Am Orthodontic Soc* 12, no. 2 (2012): 2–28; "Don't call it Early Orthodontics!" Dental Sleep Practice, November 23, 2016, https://dentalsleeppractice.com/clinician-spotlight/dont-call-early-orthodontics.

13   "New CDC report: More than 100 million Americans have diabetes or prediabetes," Centers for Disease Control and Prevention, July 18, 2017, https://www.cdc.gov/media/releases/2017/p0718-diabetes-report.html.

What's the significance of today's smaller faces? As the upper and lower jaws get smaller, so do the airways. The nasal airway is smaller and more easily obstructed. The smaller upper jaw can "trap" the lower jaw, causing it to move backward, resulting in a smaller oropharyngeal airway. We will address this phenomenon later in Chapter 5. As we have previously stated, the brain tries to figure out how to position the head to maintain the largest airway. The adaptive posture can cause muscle strain and nerve compression. When the nerves are compressed, pain is more likely. Basically, when the whole structure of the face gets smaller, everything that needs to fit into the structure is compromised. Unfortunately, there's a significant difference in the size of the face today compared to what it should be.

Dr. Weston Price is well known for his research into facial development. He spent time observing aboriginal tribes and what happened as their diets changed and processed food was introduced. He wrote a book, *Nutrition and Physical Degeneration*, which contains what even today are considered groundbreaking thoughts. The core of his thought process is the effect refined sugar has on facial development. That book has spurred other individuals—including colleagues of ours—to investigate the phenomena. We would encourage readers to investigate this on their own. It would take several volumes to outline this important subject.

"Let food be thy medicine." —HIPPOCRATES

There are a number of other negative impacts on people resulting from the combination of SAD, decreased activity, and today's overly sterile environment. There are more autoimmune disorders, asthma, and allergies in the population as a whole, including children. Interestingly, studies looking at allergies, tonsils sizes, and autoimmune diseases in kids that work on farms and around animals in less-than-sterile environments have immune systems that function normally. They don't typically end up with such health problems.[14]

This is a "double whammy." That's because the immune system is designed to defend the body against invaders; it was not designed to be idle. When everything is disinfected—antibacterial wipes are available everywhere—there are no microbes to fight, so the immune system doesn't get to do its job. When there are no pathogens for it to respond to, then the immune system begins to respond to things that are not normally pathogenic. That's why there has been an upswing in autoimmune disorders and allergies to things like peanuts, which normally shouldn't cause a reaction in the body.

The second part of the whammy is that our gastrointestinal (GI) system is an important part of our immune system. Recent medical thought is linking "leaky gut" syndrome to the ingestion of glutens and other inflammatory substances that kill off our protective gut bacteria and cause larger openings in the wall of the intestines, which then allows the larger particles to pass through the lining and invade our bodies. The larger particles include foreign proteins, as well as microorganisms that normally are not allowed to enter.[15]

When people are given the correct start as infants—breast fed, eating whole foods with little/no processed sugar, and breathing ideally—then the face develops to its genetic potential and everything works the way it is supposed to.

---

14   London School of Hygiene & Tropical Medicine, "Increase in Allergies Is Not from Being Too Clean, Just Losing Touch with 'Old Friends,' lshtm.ac.uk, October 3, 2012, https://www.lshtm.ac.uk/newsevents/news/2012/allergy_rises_not_down_to_being_too_clean__just_losing_touch_with__old_friends_.html; H. Okada, H. Feillet, and J-F Bach, "The Hygiene Hypothesis for Autoimmune and Allergic Diseases: An Update," *Clin Exp Immunol* 160, no. 1 (2010):1–9.

15   Q. Mu et al., "Leaky Gut As a Danger Signal for Autoimmune Diseases," *Frontiers in Medicine*, May 2017, https://doi.org/10.3389/fimmu.2017.00598; M. A. Odenwald and J. R. Turner, "The Intestinal Epithelial Barrier: A Therapeutic Target?" *Nature Reviews Gastroenterology and Hepatology* 14 (2017): 9–21.

The Role of Family Genetics

Starting out right means eating healthy foods and developing healthy habits. When that doesn't happen, then genetics take over as a response to a stressor—that's why family members tend to look similar. Their genetic makeup guides the body in its compensation for survival. A person may develop a very long face or a pronounced mandible (lower jaw) as a way of compensating for a narrow upper jaw that constricts the airway (since the roof of the mouth is the floor of the nose)—that is the role of genetics. There is extensive research in the field of *epigenetics*: how our genes respond to our environment.

For example, a child may regularly eat Pop-Tarts and donuts for breakfast, thinking that those are great ways to start the day. Instead, those foods are dumping sugar into their system, causing their nasal passages to become inflamed and forcing them to breathe through their mouth. That blocked nose forces the tongue posture to change, causing it to sit low in the mouth so that air can flow over it. Instead of the tip of the tongue being positioned on the soft tissue behind and just touching the top front teeth where it belongs, it is positioned behind and just touching the bottom front teeth. That will change the growth of facial structures—narrow palate and rotation of the mandible—and all of these things can cause a child to open their mouth to breathe.

When the child's mouth is open all the time, allowing him or her to breathe, the teeth don't touch as they normally would. That leads to incorrect positioning of the erupting teeth, or teeth that are coming in. During eruption, it's important for proper muscle function to be present and for the upper and lower teeth to touch intermittently, but regularly, throughout the day. This is what Dr. Ramirez-Yanez refers to when he talks about a "chewy" food diet leading to correct development of the jaw structures. If a child breathes through their mouth when their teeth are erupting, one result can be an excess area of gum above the teeth (gummy smile). That's because the upper teeth erupted more than usual due to the open mouth posture and lack of enough upper and lower tooth contact. This results in the maxilla (upper jaw) growing more vertically than is normal. The upper jaw growing downward more forces the mandible (lower jaw) to rotate down and back. The result is a longer face with a very narrow upper arch, potentially with flared top front teeth because that's where the tongue is hitting, along with a chin that looks like it's rolled back or weak. That weaker chin is a classic genetic pattern in some families.

In another family, the genetic response to the same diet may be different. When the nose gets blocked in response to excess sugar in the diet, then tongue posture drops even lower in the mouth. Instead of the tongue touching the lower front teeth, it's so low in the mouth that it touches at the gum line below the lower teeth. That actually stimulates the lower jaw to grow more forward while the upper jaw has no growth stimulus and remains underdeveloped and very small. Without the tongue applying force to the upper jaw from inside the mouth, the muscles of the upper lip and the cheeks restrain growth. The result is a face with a very forward chin but a smaller, underdeveloped upper jaw.

So genetics dictate the response to the environmental issues because families tend to behave in the same way, for example: eating sugary breakfast foods, eating sweets when they're feeling down, or simply following their traditional diet and customs. Think of an Italian grandmother telling you to "Mangia! Eat! Eat!" and presenting you with wonderful pasta dishes.

And it's harder to eat healthy today anywhere in the world, considering the SAD has pretty much permeated all of civilized society. People living in primitive areas of the world where there is still adequate food are almost better off because they're growing their own food and trapping their own protein. People in those kinds of situations actually grow and develop more along the lines of what the ideal human is supposed to look like.

Now, certain genetic predispositions also determine development. For example, the angular change from the anterior cranial base to the posterior base is essentially genetically determined. Some people have a very acute angle, others have a more obtuse angle. The more acute the angle, the more genetically predisposed a person is to having a shorter face that grows more forward. The more obtuse that angle, the longer the face tends to grow. This is part of what determines how we look—the genetic predisposition.

But again, someone who is predisposed to having a short face can still end up with a longer face if there is dysfunction, such as an obstruction in the airway, that ultimately alters the normal development of the face and mouth.

A 1981 study on rhesus monkeys found that to be true.[16] The study involved a group of monkeys that had no previous malocclusions, or malformed teeth and jaws. The monkeys were separated into groups, and those whose noses were obstructed developed different facial appearances and dental malformations—but those malocclusions developed along familial lines based on the genetics.

So, people look different based on their genetics—their familial traits—but their faces will grow in balance unless a dysfunction causes development to go awry.

---

16   E. P. Harvold et al., "Primate Experiments on Oral Respiration," *Am J Orthod* 79, no. 4 (1981): 359–72.

The Myth of the Unalterable Cranial Suture

There are twenty-two separate bones in the human skull. The majority of dentists are still taught that the suture in the brain are fused in youth. The skull is actually composed of different bones that fit together like a puzzle to create the shape of the head. Where the bones meet are sutures, or seams of fibrous tissue that connect the bones. This is partly what allows a baby's head to make it through the constricted birth canal. Traditionally, it's been taught that these seams fuse together during the teenage years to create immovable bone. However, the thought process is different in medical professions, where the theory is that those sutures remain viable or separate throughout our lives. As a person ages, the fibrous tissue gets more intricate and complex, creating dovetailing connections that, in an X-ray, appear to be solid bone.

But when seen under a microscope, it's apparent that the sutures are not solid. That means that, instead of the bones of the skull being immovable, they can actually be moved to correct dysfunctional development.

Chiropractor Mark Pick actually proved that the cranial structure is alterable through an experiment in which he stuffed a skull with dried peas. After wetting the peas and watching them expand, he found that the skull separated at the sutures to accommodate the increasing pea mass.[17]

The fact that the cranial sutures are not fused is what allows for expansion of the upper palate, or the roof of the mouth, in any age of patient. Since the roof of the mouth is the floor of the nose, expanding the patient's palate makes their internal nasal airway become broader and allows more air to get through. (See Chapters 5 and 6 for more about this treatment.)

---

17 M. G. Pick, *Cranial Sutures: Analysis, Morphology & Manipulative Strategies* (Seattle, WA: Eastland Press, 1999).

Problems of the Changing Face

When a person chronically struggles to breathe, that struggle alters the development of their face, jaws, and teeth, and a number of problems occur. These include a malformed bite, postural changes, breathing alterations, and a host of other problems.

DEVELOPMENTAL PROBLEMS THAT CAN OCCUR:

- Overbite. The top front teeth overlap the bottom front teeth.

- Underbite. The lower front teeth extend out further than the top front teeth.

- Tongue thrust. The tongue protrudes out between the front or sides of the teeth (anterior or lateral tongue thrust).

- V-shaped, narrow arch. This can cause crowding inside the mouth.

- Crowded teeth.

- Compromised facial aesthetics.

- Mouth breathing, instead of breathing through the nose, which is the proper way to breathe.

- Speech and eating difficulties.

- TMJ issues.

- Obstructive Sleep Apnea

All of these problems are the result of survival mechanisms. In trying to keep the body alive, other problems can develop that can ultimately endanger the body. For instance, when the breathing is obstructed and the mouth and tongue alter position and function, then the lips become more flaccid, and swallowing and speech can be affected. This leads to speech problems (not life threatening) or swallowing issues (could be life threatening).

Sometimes, the changes result in aesthetic issues, such as a bit of a gap between the upper front teeth. Sometimes, the upper teeth do not properly overlap the lower front teeth. The patient may feel as if their bite is fine, but the truth is that their teeth are only contacting in the back. This is referred to as an anterior open bite. While issues like an open bite may seem only aesthetic, the truth is that function is also affected.

The problem is that the body compensates for dysfunction in order to survive, which may present an aesthetic concern. Then, if the issue is fixed purely for aesthetic reasons—for instance, the person gets braces to straighten their teeth and close that gap in the front—then they are ultimately making the situation worse. The person's smile may be more attractive, and they may be able to bite down better to eat a sandwich, but without addressing the root of the problem they are actually complicating a health issue. Why? Because the problem is that they cannot breathe! They have a high arch that is crowding the tongue, which then forces the tongue lower in the mouth, which constricts the upper arch more—and the cycle goes on and on. By straightening the teeth without widening the arch, the tongue becomes more compressed or restricted. With not enough room in the mouth, the tongue is forced backward into the throat, cutting off the airway. So, from a health and survival standpoint, the patient is actually moving in the wrong direction.

The goal with any treatment is health, harmony, symmetry, and balance—something known as divine proportion (also called Phi 1:1.618). Divine proportion is essentially a geometrically calculated definition of beauty. It is found throughout nature. A healthy, high-functioning human body follows the divine proportion. When the whole body is healthier, it functions more normally and actually looks better. When the body is clicking on all cylinders, there is far less chronic pain and it's far easier to target and treat the site of an injury. But when there is dysfunction in the body, then chronic pain can lead to problems that almost never manifest at the original site of injury—the site in the body that needs to be addressed first.

CHAPTER 3

"But Doctor, It Hurts Over Here"

n our practices, we are often presented with puzzling situations. Helping people to get to the "root of their problem" is part of the challenge, and the fun of what we do.

Meredith was one of those challenging situations. She came in seeking help for pain on the left side of her face that she rated as seven on a scale of ten. She'd had been suffering with that unexplained pain for several months, and had already seen several doctors—dentists, chiropractors, and medical physicians. But none of them had been able to provide a solution. She had been diagnosed with trigeminal neuralgia and told that she would require drugs "to keep her comfortable."

At her first appointment, we began the evaluation using Motor Nerve Reflex Testing (MNRT), which is a set of neurologic tests to determine the primary site of injury. According to the MNRT, the source of her structural issue and her pain was her lower back, or sacroiliac joint (SI). She was surprised to the point of becoming upset upon hearing that diagnosis. She actually became quite insistent that the problem was in her face.

After a lot of time, and discussion, she allowed us to diagnostically apply high-intensity laser therapy to her SI joint. The treatment took about five minutes, after which she immediately sat up and, choking back tears, said, "This is the first time in seven months I can say that my face doesn't hurt!" After that demonstration, she was open to suggestions for treatment that included chiropractic care focused on the SI area. Once that therapy was completed, her treatment through our practice was much shorter.

Meredith's pains stemmed from two facts: 1) her SI joint problem was making her subconsciously grind her teeth at night, causing a lot of stress and damage to her TMJ, and 2) her entire spinal column was twisted, which ultimately caused the SI and TMJ positions to be altered. There was also a change in her posture, causing muscle strain and nerve compression and pain that was referred to her face. Once the SI issue was addressed, her posture was corrected, which stopped the clenching and took pressure off the masseter muscles of the lower jaw and the TMJ. That allowed us to successfully treat the damage that had been done to her jaw in a shorter period of time. That's usually the case with TMJ; we can treat it once the precipitating factors have been removed. That is an important concept since many other issues masquerade as TMJ/craniofacial pain issues, and TMJ issues can cause pain in other parts of the body. We must make it very clear that we did not "treat" her SI joint. It was a diagnostic experiment to determine the location of the primary injury that she was dealing with. She was referred to the correct health care professional to address the SI issue.

Chasing Symptoms

There is a lot of confusion about TMJ because there are a number of conditions that can cause facial pain that have nothing to do with the jaw joint. It's common for patients to present with pain and symptoms that actually stem from a problem in another area of the body. In fact, patients often are not even aware they have pain in the area of their body that is ultimately causing the problem. This is because of what is known as *adaptive posture*. Adaptive posture is the body's ability to protect an injured body part so it can heal. Once that injured body part is healed, posture returns to "normal." But what if the injury never heals fully? Then the adaptive posture becomes a chronic problem and causes unnatural strain on other parts of the body.

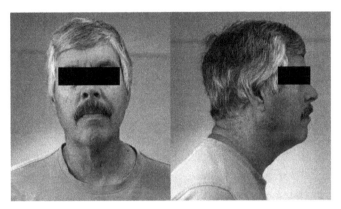

Forward head posture

The reason TMJ can be a confusing condition difficult to diagnose is because everything in the body is connected. If the jaw is out of alignment, it can cause the body to resort to the adaptive forward head posture (FHP) to open the airway. That can cause the spine to twist, and that twist will be transmitted via fascia all the way down to the toes. That's how a person with jaw pain can also have knee and foot problems. But pain can also travel in the other direction. A sore knee, foot, or hip can cause a person to assume a posture to try to protect that injury. That can create muscle strains that ultimately show up as pain in the face.

For instance, with a sore knee, every step can cause a person to unconsciously clench their teeth. Ultimately, that can cause damage to the jaw joint, a problem that needs to be treated. Although decompression therapy using an intraoral appliance will protect the jaw joint, the potential for damage will continue until the origin of the pain is addressed. In other words, until the knee pain is resolved, the muscles of the jaw will continue to get irritated every time the person takes a step. If only the symptoms are treated—in this case, the jaw pain—then the patient will never recover fully.

Diagnosing a patient's problems and determining appropriate treatment comes down to finding what's known as the primary source of pain. That may be the jaw, or it may be somewhere else in the body.

If the jaw is determined to be the primary, then treatment involves decompressing the joint and allowing the damage to heal. That treatment, however, is often misunderstood, even in the dental profession. Many practitioners do not fully comprehend the integrative nature of posture, injuries, pain, and therapies. This is why our practice is cutting edge in including providers from different professional backgrounds to help our patients achieve their optimum health. We believe that total health is a team effort.

Too often, patients are told that nothing can be done to alleviate their pain. That is because doctors who have not been able to determine the true origin of the problem simply fit the patient with a one-size-fits-all appliance in an effort to chase symptoms. But wearing a "mouth guard" for the long-term does not always address the primary cause of a problem; in some cases, it can create additional issues.

Patients who come to the office with facial pain often bring with them a collection of appliances they have received from other providers or purchased over the counter—these are the remedies that are the result of going to a provider, pointing to their jaw, and saying, "It hurts here." John Beck, an orthopedic surgeon, used to refer to this treatment model as "the dumb leading the blind."

Oral splints, for instance, are designed to separate the upper and lower teeth, protect teeth from damage, and relax the jaw muscles. Unfortunately, without any real thought put into a comprehensive treatment plan, patients often find that the splint ultimately doesn't help. That's because simply allowing the muscle to relax may not address the real problem, such as degenerative joint disease, displaced discs, or nasal airway inadequacy.

Peeling Back the Layers

For most patients, alleviating their pain is a matter of peeling back the layers. Addressing one issue often alleviates some of their pain. However, once that pain is gone, they may become aware of pain somewhere else in the body, often from an injury they didn't even know they had.

We encounter this daily, when a patient will say "my jaw feels great but my lower back is bothering me now." This is why our integrated practice model is necessary. We can address more than the jaw or the teeth.

As mentioned previously, the reason for the unusual symptom patterns is because the body compensates for injuries by altering the way it moves and operates. Those altered body postures can then create other injuries caused by moving unnaturally over a period of time.

For instance, it's not uncommon to correct an obstructed airway issue that has caused a FHP (forward head posture) only to have the patient then report that they have pain in the foot. The reason is that the FHP position shifts all the body weight forward, which causes the body to alter its normal posture, placing more pressure and weight on the ball of the foot while walking. Once the airway obstruction is removed and the body moves upright, then the patient may notice that their foot hurts less because the previous strain was removed. The injury was the result of the pressure that was placed upon the peroneal nerve in the lower portion of the leg, causing inflammation, while compensating for the FHP.

Healthy Body

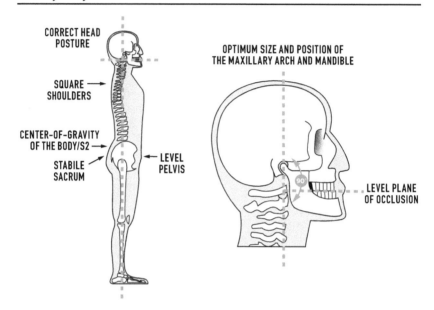

CORRECT HEAD POSTURE

SQUARE SHOULDERS

CENTER-OF-GRAVITY OF THE BODY/S2

STABILE SACRUM

LEVEL PELVIS

OPTIMUM SIZE AND POSITION OF THE MAXILLARY ARCH AND MANDIBLE

90

LEVEL PLANE OF OCCLUSION

Unhealthy Body

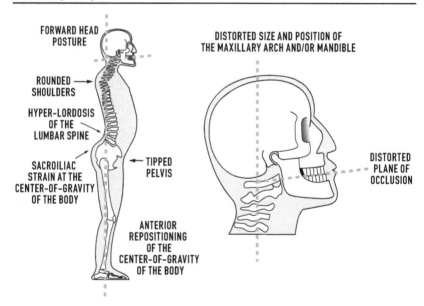

FORWARD HEAD POSTURE

ROUNDED SHOULDERS

HYPER-LORDOSIS OF THE LUMBAR SPINE

SACROILIAC STRAIN AT THE CENTER-OF-GRAVITY OF THE BODY

TIPPED PELVIS

ANTERIOR REPOSITIONING OF THE CENTER-OF-GRAVITY OF THE BODY

DISTORTED SIZE AND POSITION OF THE MAXILLARY ARCH AND/OR MANDIBLE

DISTORTED PLANE OF OCCLUSION

---

18   James E. Carlson, Physiologic Occlusion (2004).

The same can be true with a TMJ joint. As the injured joint heals, the brain alters compensating posture in an attempt to protect other areas of the body. Staci, for instance, began feeling great very soon after receiving her custom-made appliance for TMJ. Then, a couple of weeks later, she started experiencing pain in other areas of her body. An examination at that point revealed that she had an injury in her left foot that needed to be addressed. That meant adjusting her treatment plan to include a referral to a chiropractor to address the foot injury.

Remember: The brain's primary drive is to keep the body breathing and upright. With every movement and every step, the brain makes calculations to ensure that the body keeps functioning. Walking on a nice, level surface makes it easier for the brain to calculate what the body needs to breathe and stay upright. But on a gravelly, bumpy, and treacherous path, the brain has to work harder, and more adaptations need to be made. With every change the body makes, the brain recalculates.

When treatment corrects an injury, it changes the rules—it changes the brain's game plan, so to speak. That forces the brain to figure out new ways to compensate, potentially causing pain in another area. Addressing that pain makes the brain compensate again, which may cause pain to show up in another area. That's what it means to address pain one layer at a time. Ultimately, the brain is prioritizing pain—it's trying to figure out what the next worst injury or primary injury will be. If that primary injury was originally TMJ, but the TMJ is addressed, then the brain eliminates the TMJ as a concern and changes the body's posture to address the next priority. If there's another area of the body that has enough damage to draw the brain's attention, then it will make new postural compensations to address that injury. Usually, that secondary area of pain on its own would have required postural compensation if the TMJ hadn't been classified as more important.

The brain makes postural compensations for only one thing at a time, and that is whatever is most urgent or the greatest threat to survival.

Take the case of Tony, a sixty-four-year-old male whose chief concern was pain in his jaw. During our initial conversation, he mentioned that he was scheduled for knee replacement surgery in two months. He was unable to climb a set of stairs without great difficulty and pain. I advised him that those symptoms might change—it would be fun to see. We did a home sleep test and he received a physician's diagnosis of Obstructive Sleep Apnea (OSA). He went forward with a daytime TMJ orthotic and nighttime, FDA-approved appliance for OSA. After three months of therapy, he reported that he had no issues climbing stairs and no pain in his knees or jaw, so he had cancelled his surgery. His difficulty breathing had caused forward head posture, which caused strain on his knees, which then began to hurt, causing him to clench his jaw, which then caused his jaw pain. Once we restored his nasal airway so he could breathe at night, corrected his adaptive posture, and stopped his clenching—his symptoms resolved! Stairs were no longer an issue!

Chronic Pain—the Great Deceiver

It's surprising for many patients to find a dentist discovering problems in other areas of the body. For instance, when a patient is fitted with an oral appliance to address their TMJ, and then their foot begins to cause them pain, they sometimes point to their TMJ treatment as the source of the problem. But again, the new pain is usually a secondary issue moving into the primary position, since the primary problem—the TMJ—was addressed.

When patients come in for treatment, we listen to their issues to get an understanding of where they're feeling pain. Then, regardless of what they identify as the location of their pain, we do a comprehensive evaluation to locate the true source—we let their body, specifically their brain, tell us what is really wrong, in spite of where the patient says it hurts. We often act as the team quarterback, helping direct treatment.

Treating the symptoms based solely on the patient's description is an unfortunate trap that many physicians fall into—they assume that where the patient is pointing is the source of the pain. We listen, but then we follow a protocol that builds one piece of information on top of another until the clear primary source of pain is evident. That's how we find out when jaw pain is actually being caused by a foot injury—and vice versa. On some level, every time a patient comes to the office, they really are a different patient.

The doctor who developed the tests that we use to identify the primary source of pain is an orthopedic surgeon, John Beck. He understood that chronic pain is different than acute pain.[19] Acute pain is what a person experiences when they, for instance, fall off a ladder and land on their knee, causing their knee to be banged up and swollen. They go see a doctor, point to their knee, and explain what happened. The doctor listens to their story, examines the knee, and determines that, yes, the pain and swelling is from falling off a ladder. Then the doctor treats the knee, and the treatment is successful.

Diagnosing and treating chronic pain is completely different. Let's look at the same scenario: A person falls off a ladder and injures their knee. They hate going to doctors, so they "shake it off," and eventually the knee seems to get better. In reality, it doesn't heal properly, but because their body made the necessary compensations for the injury, the swelling goes down and the knee no longer seems to ache or be causing pain.

---

19   John L. Beck, "Practical Application of Neuropostural Evaluations, the P.A.N.E. Process: Basic Principles and the First Three Tests," *Practical Pain Management* 8, no. 7 (September 2008): 47–53.

What has happened is that the brain (because it is concerned more about loss of function than it is about pain) begins to make postural changes to compensate for the injured knee. That postural compensation places additional demand on other structures, which may begin to break down. Once the brain senses that survival is threatened, the body is put into that sympathetic, fight-or-flight state discussed in Chapter 1.

Now, the knee doesn't appear to hurt, but the patient starts having lower back pain. He goes to the doctor, who listens to him describe his lower back pain. Since the patient doesn't connect the lower back pain to the hurt knee resulting from the fall off the ladder, the knee and fall are never mentioned to the doctor. The doctor takes a look at the patient's lower back, which according to the patient is the source of the pain and recognizes that the hips are canted (angled) and the spinal column is curved. The diagnosis is scoliosis, and the solution, it appears, is to adjust the spine to straighten the hips—problem solved. Or so they think.

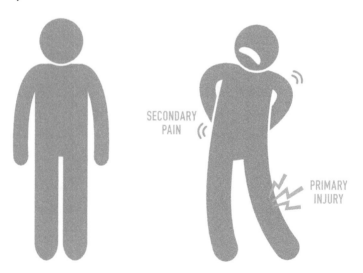

However, what's really going on is that, in compensating for the hurt knee, the brain has forced the body to shift the way it normally would move. That has forced the spinal column to twist in an unnatural way, all because the body is trying to protect the knee. As soon as the patient steps off the doctor's treatment table and takes one step on the leg with the bad knee, everything shifts again, throwing the hips and spine out of alignment.

Everything the doctor did was for naught because they were addressing the problems out of the proper order. The primary source of the patient's problem is not identified as the injured knee. The way to heal chronic pain is to address the structural problems in the order that the brain prioritizes. We often tell patients that it is like telling your child you want to shampoo their bedroom carpet, but it is littered with toys and clothes. The correct sequence of events is to pick up the clothes, vacuum the carpet, and then shampoo it. No sane person would try to shampoo the carpet first, because we all recognize it will not work.

Darla is a good example of what it means to address each primary issue in order. She came in complaining of joint pain and, through a comprehensive evaluation, it was determined that her TMJ was the primary. An orthotic alleviated her jaw pain, but then she began to complain of pain in her foot. She came back pointing to the appliance as the culprit for her foot pain. Testing revealed that, with the orthotic in place, her foot was shown to be the primary injury. When she removed the appliance, testing revealed that her jaw was the primary injury. While the appliance was in, her brain decided that the jaw was good to go, and then it looked for some other injury that was significant enough to keep her in a sympathetic state. At that point, the appropriate recommendation was for her to be referred to a physician who could treat her foot. The instructions

> The way to heal chronic pain is to address the structural problems in the order that the brain prioritizes.

were given for her to wear her oral orthotic while seeking treatment for her foot.

Darla's is a good example of how chronic pain is deceiving. It may occur in areas that seem completely unrelated to the primary source of pain. It demonstrates how we must address each structural problem in the correct order and how that order may change as treatment progresses.

Clenching, in particular, can cause chronic pain in other areas. Clenching traumatizes the jaw joint, but it also causes pain, such as headaches, shoulder aches, neck aches, and more due to muscle fatigue and damage to structures. Some patients report clenching during the day, but they don't realize that they're also clenching at night. And nighttime clenching is far more intense than daytime clenching. Yet, the primary way to resolve clenching is often to correct an obstructed nasal airway and to reduce the abnormally high blood CO_2 levels. The increase in blood CO_2 levels may cause the masseter muscle to contract, causing "clenching," and it might be very painful.

Again, it's all about peeling back the layers. Some patients, especially those who have had issues for a long time, may have several areas that have been compromised by a primary injury. That requires treatment to go in a specific order as the brain decides what issue is worse, meaning that a series of issues will become primary as each is addressed along the way.

Some of those primary injuries may have to be addressed by other health care providers, which was the case with Darla. She was referred to a podiatrist for the problem with her foot. This again demonstrates the importance of a health team to address our patients' needs.

Ultimately, although the patient can share what areas of their body are in pain, testing reveals where the real problems are—and they may be one after another until they're all resolved.

CHAPTER 4

TMJ and Sleep Apnea—
A Real Combo

G eorge was in his seventies when he came in wanting to be fitted with an oral appliance to address his sleep apnea. He had already been diagnosed by a sleep physician, so we were happy to oblige his request.

During the detailed initial examination, he also reported that he had neck and back pain. No wonder, considering that he had a forward head posture of more than five inches. Based on laws of physics and biomechanics, in that position, his normal fifteen-pound head had a relative weight of seventy-five pounds.

During the intraoral examination, we also found that the partial denture he was wearing to replace of all of his lower molars was completely worn out. He was "overclosing." In other words, his lower jaw needed to move upward to compensate for his worn teeth. If you were to measure two points (one on his nose and one on his chin) in a vertical dimension, you would see that they had moved closer together. The result is the shortening of the masseter and temporalis muscles, creating pain. It also constricts his airway, causing forward head posture.

At the time, he reported that he was already seeing a physical therapist to help "correct his posture," as he described it, but he had not seen much improvement.

To demonstrate to George how the treatment we offered could help him, we corrected his jaw position using tongue blades. This corrected the vertical dimension he had lost. Almost immediately, he raised his head four inches, nearly correcting his posture. That simple act reduced the relative weight of his head to about thirty-five pounds. The evaluation included before-and-after photos of his posture, and he was amazed to see the difference such a small change could make.

We referred him to a general dentist who understands our protocols and who could fit George with a new partial denture to help his posture. George left the office with a spring in his step—he was so excited to find answers to the problems that had plagued him for some time.

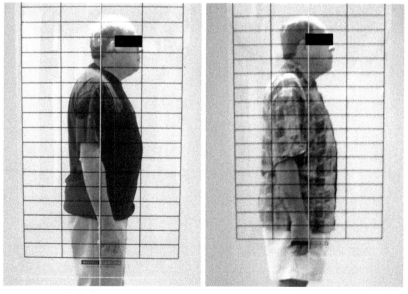

Before treatment   After treatment

TMJ—A Complicated Joint

TMJ is a dysfunction of the temporomandibular joint, or the jaw joints. The TMJ is the most complicated joint in the body. It is distinctive because there are two joints connected by a single rigid bone. It is also distinctive in the way that it moves—it rotates and then slides to open fully without dislocating.

There are a number of dysfunctions that affect the TMJ. These are broken down into two groups: intracapsular and extracapsular.

Intracapsular involves dysfunction occurring within the joint capsule. The joint capsule is composed of fibrous tissue that holds the joint together and keeps it protected from bacteria and infection. The capsule contains a disc, ligaments, the condyle (rounded end of the mandible, or lower bone of the jaw), and the fossa, which is basically the "socket" at the base of the skull bone that the condyle fits into.

If the disc is in its correct position in relation to the condyle and fossa (basically in between where the two bones meet), and if all the ligaments are healthy, then the joint functions beautifully. If the ligaments get damaged or the disc gets displaced, or if both damage and displacement occur, then the joint can start breaking down. That displacement can happen from a macrotrauma, such as a blow to the jaw from an accident, or from a microtrauma, which is what occurs when a person clenches and grinds their teeth. TMJ is an orthopedic issue within the joint that occurs because the joint starts breaking down.

Extracapsular refers to problems occurring outside the capsule, most commonly involving a muscular dysfunction. Again, if someone is constantly clenching their teeth because of a problem in their knee, the muscles associated with the TMJ will get sore and create symptoms, but the actual jaw joint capsule and all that it contains may be relatively healthy.

There can also be combination intracapsular and extracapsular dysfunctions when it comes to TMJ. Once the joint starts breaking down, the muscles have to work harder to protect the joint. To do that, they'll resort to what's known as muscle splinting or spasms, which is when the muscles become stiff to prevent them from being used.

Part of diagnosing TMJ is a matter of trying to discern whether the problem is inside or outside the joint. Once the diagnosis is made, then the appropriate treatments are provided.

SYMPTOMS OF TMJ

When a body part is injured, the muscles that surround it work very hard to support and protect the injured structure. This is referred to as "muscle splinting." Again, the brain is constantly making calculations to accommodate the injury, causing different areas of the body to work overtime. At some point, they get exhausted from all the extra effort, or a nerve gets compressed and that results in pain. Plus, there's compression inside the joint, which directly affects nerves located in the joint. When inflammation and swelling are present, edema (swelling caused by fluid retention) can create pressure and pain. Those are just a couple of ways pain is created—there are many other reasons that areas of the body can experience pain.

COMMON SYMPTOMS OF TMJ/TMD

- ✔ Facial pain
- ✔ Jaw pain
- ✔ Headaches
- ✔ Neck pain
- ✔ Back pain
- ✔ Shoulder pain
- ✔ Inability to open the mouth
- ✔ Noises (clicking) upon opening and closing the mouth
- ✔ Abnormal jaw movement

With TMJ, that pain can manifest in the face, jaw, neck, shoulders, or back. Other TMJ symptoms can also include a clicking, popping, or grating sound when the joint is used. The joint may also "freeze" to the point that the range of motion in the jaw is limited. These occur because of internal derangement of the joint involving either a displaced disc, a dislocated jaw, rubbing bone on bone, or an injury to the condyle.

That happened to Joey, a fourteen-year-old patient who came in with a chief complaint of jaw popping when he chewed that was so loud other members of the family refused to eat dinner with him at the table. Testing indicated that he had Morton's neuroma, which is a thickening of the tissue around a nerve in the foot between the toes that produces a sharp, burning pain in the ball of the foot. When the foot was identified as the primary, a couple of efforts produced a temporary solution in just a manner of minutes. The first effort, a toe spacer, did not resolve his problem, but shimming his arches immediately silenced the noise. That meant the solution for Joey's primary was a referral to a local podiatrist for corrective foot orthotics. He and his father were incredulous until I kept removing and replacing the "foot splints" and the noises predictably would disappear or recur.

There are also a number of less-common symptoms of TMJ. These are usually neuromuscular in origin.

If the jaw is in an abnormal position, it's basically been dislocated. Any TMJ that is making noise is dislocated. I often ask patients if they would tolerate a knee or elbow making those kinds of sounds and the answer is usually a resounding *no!* When dislocation happens, all the muscles in the face that help control the movement of the jaw—the temporalis and masseters (the mandibular elevators), the suprahyoids and the pterygoids—try to balance the jaw as best they can to avoid the neurologic input to the brain that's screaming "pain, pain, pain."

When they have to compensate, they work really hard and that causes them to cramp up—that's where the pain comes from. These cramps or muscle spasms can cause some very interesting symptoms.

UNCOMMON SYMPTOMS OF TMJ/TMD

- ✗ Inability to swallow
- ✗ Vomiting—upon turning to the right
- ✗ Visual problems
- ✗ Numbness of the hands
- ✗ Movement disorder—tics/twitches
- ✗ Burning tongue

The cramping also causes the muscles to function abnormally, and there is more involved than just the muscles surrounding the jaw joint. The muscles of the neck can also be affected, including the trapezius (down the back), the sternocleidomastoid muscle (alongside the neck), the suprahyoid (under the chin), and the infrahyoid (down the front of the neck). These muscles help position the head and prevent it from tipping too far forward or backward. Even the oropharyngeal muscles (in the throat) don't work properly when they're tired and overworked. That can make it difficult to swallow.

Claire, for instance, was one patient whose oropharyngeal muscles were in spasm to the point that, when she ate, the food went up her nose instead of down her throat. Her swallowing mechanism was essentially working backward because the muscles were so injured and out of control. There also was involvement of the vagus nerve. Stabilization and support of her mandible caused a reversal of symptoms. She was unable to wean successfully from her orthotics and needed to have Phase II orthodontic treatment to actually change her orofacial structures to stabilize her result.

Vomiting is another uncommon symptom of TMJ, caused by an

injured vagus nerve, which runs through the same area of the neck and face. Sandy entered our practice with her chief concern being that she vomited every time she turned her head to the right. She was TMJ primary and elected to proceed with treatment. Decompression of her jaw joint using an oral appliance stopped her chronic vomiting within a week.

For a small percentage of patients, visual problems can also indicate TMJ because the base of the eyeball socket is the maxilla (the upper jaw). When TMJ causes distortion of the cranium, or the skull, then the eyeball can get actually get squeezed in the process, which changes the shape of the lens. That causes visual disturbance. The good news is that when the cranium is normalized by appliance therapy, then the visual disturbance often goes away. Once again, we are treating the TMJ problem and see unusual and beneficial side effects.

TMJ often can contribute to movement disorders such as ticks and twitching, numbness in an extremity such as the hands, and even a burning sensation in the tongue. These are all related to a structure called the subnucleus caudalis in the neck, which is the site of four cranial nerves—oculomotor, facial, glossopharyngeal, and vagus. This is the only place in the body where those nerves reside in close proximity to one another. These nerves stimulate various areas of the body, including the eyes (oculomotor); face (facial); tongue, throat, tonsils, and ears (glossopharyngeal); and stomach (vagus). When these nerves are injured, they can become overly stimulated and cause abnormal behaviors or symptoms.

For instance, the tongue is innervated by three of the four nerves. When a person experiences a condition known as "burning tongue," which is when the entire tongue feels like it's on fire, then that means three pairs of those cranial nerves are being stimulated at the same time. Burning tongue has been traditionally treated with topical medications to address a microbial infection. I have successfully treated many people with "burning tongue."

Again, these nerves reside in the neck. A jaw joint out of alignment to the point that breathing is affected may result in improper breathing and ultimately an adaptive forward head posture. That abnormal neck posture causes excessive muscle tension or rotation of vertebrae, resulting in compression of those nerves. That causes them to fire or behave abnormally, leading to those movement disorders, numbness, or burning tongue. We have seen improvement in multiple patients with movement disorders. Once again, we are not treating Parkinson's disease or ticks. We are treating TMJ disorders and seeing beneficial side effects.

Patients often don't even realize that these uncommon symptoms are caused by their TMJ until after they've been treated and their symptoms are relieved.

Sleep Apnea—Snoring and More

At some level, TMJ and sleep apnea go hand in hand. In fact, one study of patients found that more than half of those with sleep apnea also had symptoms of TMJ.[20]

Apnea refers to pauses in breathing for more than ten seconds, one or more times during sleep. Each of those pauses can last from ten seconds to minutes. Those lapses can be caused by a collapse of the airway during sleep, nasal obstruction, soft palate interference, or the tongue falling backward to block the airway. When that happens, the muscles of the jaw move in a manner designed to open the airway. Sometimes the teeth get in the way, which leads to bruxism or grinding of the teeth. That bruxing creates repeated stress on the jaw joint, and

---

20   P. A. Cunali et al., "Prevalence of Temporomandibular Disorders in Obstructive Sleep Apnea Patients Referred for Oral Appliance Therapy," *Journal of Oral & Facial Pain and Headache* 23, no. 4 (2009): 339–44.

ultimately causes symptoms of TMJ. The increased levels of CO_2 in the blood also cause contraction of the masseter muscles, causing muscular pain and damage to the teeth.

There are three types of sleep apnea: central, obstructive, and mixed (both central and obstructive). With central sleep apnea, the brain simply forgets to breathe. It is a neurologic disorder and the only solution is a continuous positive airway pressure (CPAP) machine.

Obstructive sleep apnea (OSA) is what the name implies. Something gets in the way of your breathing, whether it's your tongue, a clogged nose, or something else in the airway from the tip of the nose to the throat. The four most common obstructors are: a clogged nose, soft palate, the tongue, or the airway itself collapses. While a CPAP machine is often used for OSA, there are also other types of treatment. Those treatments will be discussed in the chapters to follow.

The real problem with sleep apnea is that the pauses in breathing can lead to a drop-in oxygen levels in the blood. Anything below 90 percent oxygenation can begin to deprive the brain and body of the oxygen it needs to function well.

COMMON SIGNS AND SYMPTOMS OF SLEEP APNEA IN ADULTS

- ✔ Snoring
- ✔ Gasping for breath
- ✔ Daytime sleepiness
- ✔ Fatigue
- ✔ Depression
- ✔ Chronic pain

Snoring occurs when the tissues in the mouth—the soft palate (roof), tongue, and throat—relax as a person falls into Stage 3 of sleep. When the tissues relax enough that they block the airway, the airflow causes the tissues to vibrate. The narrower the airway, the more vibration, which means a louder snore.

Gasping for breath. Rather than the sleep apnea sufferer recognizing this in themselves, jerking awake and gasping for breath is usually witnessed by a bed partner. That happens when the brain causes a person to rouse in an effort to restore breathing.

Daytime sleepiness is one of the most common symptoms of sleep apnea. Someone who is tired or fatigued all the time, or who always seems to be sapped of energy, may be experiencing sleep apnea. Daytime sleepiness means falling asleep inappropriately while driving or at a stoplight, needing a nap after lunch, or dozing off at work.

Fatigue is reported more frequently in females rather than males. It is the inability to "get up and go," or a general feeling of exhaustion. People often say they feel sapped of all their energy.

Depression is another symptom of disrupted sleep—and that can actually go both ways. Depression can cause sleep disruptions, and sleep disruptions can cause depression. That seems only natural— anyone whose sleep is being disrupted from five to one hundred times an hour is never really going to be well rested. That can cause depression and anxiety. These issues are why we work closely with psychiatrists and psychologists.

Anxiety is often seen in conjunction with chronic pain and disturbed sleep. Our breathing reeducation program is one way to address this and help you decrease your medications.

Chronic pain. Like depression, chronic pain (another symptom) can be a two-way street. Anyone in chronic pain is going to have trouble sleeping, and without good sleep, their body will start to have aches and pains.

One patient, an elderly gentleman, had lingering shoulder pain after surgery, and he was forced to sleep on his back the entire night—

if he rolled onto his shoulder, the pain would wake him. Sleeping in one position without the ability to move around as needed can certainly keep a person from getting a good night's rest. And in his case, trying to get comfortable only made the situation worse.

Hormone disruption. Sleep disturbances disrupt the body's ability to properly produce the hormones it needs to function and grow. For instance, in Stage 3 sleep, the body produces human growth hormones (HGH), also known as somatotropin. HGH stimulates growth and cell reproduction and regeneration, and it plays an important role in metabolism. HGH levels in the blood change throughout the day and are affected by stress, diet, exercise, and sleep. During sleep at night, HGH helps repair cell damage that has occurred during the day. If sleep is constantly interrupted, then instead of the body's cells getting repaired, they continue to break down, resulting in more and more pain.

Over time, disrupted sleep can even lead to potentially deadly diseases. A study conducted by the University of Chicago found that fragmented sleep can impede the immune system's ability to do its job, which can raise the risk of some cancers and potentially allow existing tumors to grow at an accelerated rate.[21] Women often get poor sleep as they enter menopause.

Frequent need to urinate at night, known as *nocturia*, is also a sign of sleep apnea. While some patients actually do suffer from an overactive bladder that causes them to urinate almost hourly during the day, others have grown accustomed to getting up multiple times a night to go to the bathroom. But frequent need to urinate overnight is often a sign of sleep apnea. That's because during Stage 3 sleep, the body usually releases antidiuretic hormone (ADH), which prevents fluid

---

21   J. Easton, "Fragmented Sleep Accelerates Cancer Growth," University of Chicago, news release, January 27, 2014, https://news.uchicago.edu/article/2014/01/27/ fragmented-sleep-accelerates-cancer-growth.

from filling the bladder. However, sleep apnea interrupts Stage 3 sleep and alters the release of ADH, causing more urine to be produced and fill the bladder. That triggers the person to wake and head for the bathroom.

In fact, one of the benchmarks that helps determine whether a patient's apnea is effectively being addressed is the number of times a night they get up to go to the bathroom.

> One of the benchmarks that helps determine whether a patient's apnea is effectively being addressed is the number of times a night they get up to go to the bathroom.

SLEEP APNEA IN CHILDREN

While children experience many of the same symptoms as adults, they also struggle with additional problems from lack of sleep.

Bedwetting. Although adults with sleep apnea may struggle to get through a night without a trip to the bathroom, when ADH production is disrupted in children because of sleep apnea, they often end up wetting the bed. (The same holds true for adults who lack bladder control.) Studies have shown that improving airways can reduce nighttime eneuresis (bedwetting) up to 80 percent.[22]

Hyperactivity, pseudo-ADHD, learning disabilities, anxiety, and depression are all potential symptoms of sleep apnea in children. These conditions can be related to sleep disruption and hyperventilation during mouth breathing. It's terrifying what happens to children who suffer from sleep apnea—so much so that it's quickly becoming a top priority for us to educate parents and caregivers about the subject.[23]

Imagine how much an adult gets done during the day when

---

22   L. J. Brooks and H. I. Topol, "Enuresis in Children with Sleep Apnea," *JPediatr* 142, no. 5 (May 2003): 515–18.

23   N. A. Youssef et al., "Is Obstructive Sleep Apnea Associated with ADHAD?" *Annal Clin Psychiatry* 23, no. 3 (Aug 2011): 213–24.

they're suffering from sleep apnea. If you've been up all night, or had your sleep interrupted several times a minute, how alert do you really think you'd be? Well, it's no different for kids. As discussed in Chapter 1, children with sleep apnea are often misdiagnosed as having behavioral problems, such as ADHD, and then are prescribed some kind of medication. They even may be labeled as having learning disorders! We've seen this in children as young as age three! But again, lack of sleep leads to changes in the brain.

As mentioned in Chapter 1, in children, sleep disruptions can lead to permanent brain changes. Those occur in two areas of the brain related to learning: 1) the hippocampus, which is located in the temporal lobe (the sides of the brain), which is where learning and memory storage occur; and 2) the right frontal cortex, which oversees executive function, or the ability to access and use memory. These changes occur because oxygen deprivation and fragmented sleep alter the brain's chemistry, and lead to the poor development of neurons, the brain's communicators. Children with OSA have been found to have mean IQ test scores as much as fifteen points lower than children without OSA.[24]

In children, enlarged tonsils and adenoids often cause an obstructed airway, so surgical removal can often remove the obstruction and lead to better sleep. Research and our experience has found that this surgery may not be optimally effective.

Creating a Good Environment for Sleep

Part of the challenge in diagnosing and treating sleep apnea is that a number of things can affect sleep. Everyone knows what it means to toss and turn now and then. But when a person loses sleep night after night, then the matter needs further investigation. And the cause is

---

24   Johns Hopkins Medical Institutions, "Childhood Sleep Apnea Linked To Brain Damage, Lower IQ," Science Daily, August 27, 2006, accessed November 17, 2017, https://www. sciencedaily.com/releases/2006/08/060826171825.htm."

not always sleep apnea.

For some patients, getting a good night's sleep is a matter of locking their pet out of the bedroom. For others, it's simply a matter of clearing their mind by giving thanks for all the good that's happened to them.

However, for some people, there's something a little more emotional or mentally unsettling going on. Sometimes, those issues linger so long that it means a referral to a psychologist or a counselor of some sort.

A number of other factors can cause sleep disturbances and addressing these is a matter of dealing with what's known as "sleep hygiene," or creating a good environment for sleep. Since the bedroom should be reserved for sleep and "hanky-panky" only, then here are a few tips for getting a better night's sleep.

Sleep Hygiene Tips

Keep it quiet. Chances are, anyone living next to the L-train in Chicago is going to have a little trouble sleeping. Ideally, the bedroom should be a place of silence. That means no TV, no ticking clocks, no smartphone beeping out endless notifications. If outside noises can't be prevented, then consider purchasing earplugs or a machine that produces white noise—such as a room fan or a sleep machine.

Douse the lights. The body needs darkness to regenerate. That's because of the circadian rhythm, an internal "clock" of the body's sleep/wake cycles. The circadian rhythm tends to follow the cycle of day and night, which is one reason why it can be tougher to stay awake in the winter months when the days are shorter. To promote a more regular cycle, it's important to have a bedroom that is cool and dark—void of lights. Block out lights from outside the room with room-darkening shades. And cover or remove lights in the room that can disrupt sleep. From alarm clocks to TVs to nightlights, even the green lights on smoke alarms, turn off or cover the lights for a better night's sleep.[25]

Clean up the clutter. Clutter can be distracting, keeping your mind awake when all you want to do is sleep. Remove papers and other clutter that has nothing to do with getting some rest. Using a journal to write down all the things you are trying to remember prior to sleeping reduces the clutter in your brain.

Eat in the dining room—not the bed. Avoid eating food in bed. In fact, avoid eating anything heavy or stimulating for several hours before going to bed.

Work in the office—not the bedroom. Avoid doing work in bed as well. No reading emails, no reading of any sort. The goal is for your mind to be ready to rest when your head hits the pillow.

No caffeine or alcohol. Caffeine—even decaffeinated—can stay in your body for hours, so be sure to have the last caffeinated drink of the day early in the afternoon. And contrary to popular belief, alcohol doesn't help you sleep—in moderate amounts, it's a stimulant. Red wine also increases the inflammation of nasal tissue, causing your nose to be more blocked (think snoring). Avoid that nightcap before heading off to sleep.

Take a bath. A drop in body temperature can induce sleep. Take a nice, warm bath or shower an hour before bedtime, and as your body temperature lowers, you'll fall asleep more easily. Using Epsom salts in your bath prior to bedtime will also aid sleep by acting as a muscle relaxant.

Comfort. Sleep is so much easier when you have a comfortable mattress, an appropriate pillow, and soft, clean sheets.

---

25 Harvard Medical School, "Blue Light Has a Dark Side," *Harvard Health Letter*, Dec 30, 2017, www.health.harvard.edu/staying-healthy/blue-light-has-a-dark-side; J. F. Duffy and C. A. Czeisler, "Effect of Light on Human Circadian Physiology," *Sleep Med Clin* 4, no. 2 (Jun 2009): 165–77.

Keep it timely. Avoid naps and try to form a regular routine of when you go to bed and when you wake up—even on weekends and your days off.

When it comes to getting a good night's sleep, good sleep hygiene is often the best medicine.

Diagnosing Airway Obstruction

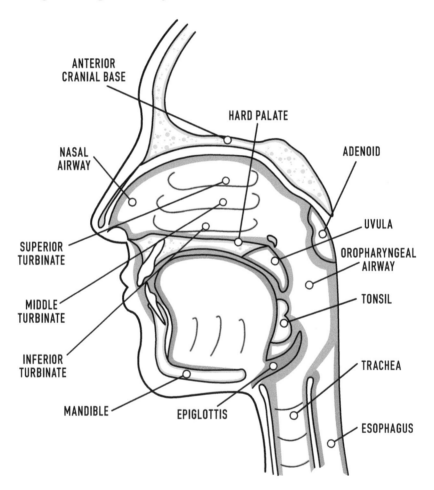

In diagnosing and treating the most likely areas of obstruction, we look at four major areas: the nose or nasal airway, the soft palate (the roof of the mouth toward the back), the tongue, and the oropharyngeal walls, which are the fleshy areas at the back of the throat. Any of these areas can relax during sleep, and then collapse in on the airway and cause an obstruction.

While we can treat sleep apnea with oral appliances, diagnosing it can only be done by a sleep physician (DO, MD) following a sleep study. There are two types of sleep studies: hospital-based (a polysomnography, or PSG) and home-based (home sleep testing, or HST).

The hospital-based test is best for children or adults who are borderline, and anyone with a severe medical problem that might endanger their health. A home-based test is fairly accurate, but it's not as sensitive as a hospital-based test. That's why hospital-based tests are better for patients who are borderline, because home-based tests may report normal results even if there is a sleep apnea issue. Home-based tests can have a great amount of variability—we've seen two-night home-based tests return results that were as much as 10 points different because breathing at night can vary significantly night to night. Sometimes it can be a daytime activity that affects how we sleep at night. In-lab studies (PSG) are more expensive and people often are uncomfortable with the wire leads and the concept of someone "watching them sleep."

In our practice, all of our patients are evaluated for both TMJ and sleep apnea, because some have TMJ only, some only have sleep disorders, and some have both. An accurate diagnosis—determining the exact position the jaw needs to be in—is the key to successful treatment. That's what happens in Phase I. We have found in our practice that the comorbidity is 50 percent. In other words, 50 percent of the people who come in for "jaw pain" have sleep apnea and 50 percent of the people referred by a medical physician for OSA oral appliance therapy have an underlying TMJ disorder.

CHAPTER 5

Phase I TMJ Treatment

D r. Lynn's practice, the TMJ and Sleep Therapy Centre of Chicago, specializes in Phase I of TMJ treatment. In this area of the practice, only those cases that are nearly assured an exceptional outcome are treated. This is due to our use of neurologic testing to screen our patients so we only treat those people whom it is correct to treat. But there are so many stories about patient success, it's hard to really choose one.

Perhaps the most impressive was LaDona, a female in her twenties who had daily migraine headaches along with many other issues indicating a lot of inflammation, including chronic knee injuries, polycystic ovarian disease, and asthma.

After undergoing a comprehensive evaluation and having a treatment plan customized to her needs, she came in to get her appliances and begin treatment. We were running behind on our schedule so an assistant delivered the appliances, and LaDona left to run a thirty-minute errand. When she returned to the practice to complete the day's appointment—verification that the appliance fit, along with a round of laser therapy—she reported that her migraine had already disappeared! For the first time in months, her head didn't feel like it was going to explode. Even better, her migraines never returned. She successfully completed Phase I treatment and it made a huge impact on the quality of her life.

The Goal of Phase I Treatment

The jaw joint is the only joint in the body that has another structure outside the joint that determines one of its limits of motion. That outside structure is the teeth. The teeth are influential in how the jaw sits, especially when the mouth is closed. It is normal for teeth to touch intermittently day and night, but for the most part, in a resting position, they are slightly apart when the mouth is closed. It is estimated that the total time teeth are in contact while awake is twenty minutes daily. Even though they are apart most of the time while awake, the teeth determine how much damage the jaw joint sustains. Very worn-down teeth allow the jaw joint to over-seat and strain all the ligaments that are trying keep the joint alignment correct. This is true especially in people who brux or grind their teeth.

Ligaments are more like ropes than they are like rubber bands. When they start getting strained, they begin to distort, fray, and can even tear. When that happens, the landing point for the teeth—the point at which they touch—can only be positioned as ideally as possible with an appliance.

That correct position is three-dimensional, ensuring that the bite moves correctly side to side, back and forth, and up and down. We refer to the three planes as: cant, A-P, and rotation. A pilot would describe them as pitch, roll, and yaw. The correction is customized based upon patient need. For instance, one patient may need the jaw to be opened one millimeters on one side, while the other side may need a three-millimeter correction to align the jaw. Or the correction may be rotational—one side may be farther back than the other, so the entire jaw may need to be rotated slightly.

Phase I treatment addresses these corrections while allowing the joint to heal. *Phase I does not move teeth.* Per the guidelines published by the American Academy of Craniofacial Pain and the American Academy of Orofacial Pain, Phase I treatment does not make any permanent changes. We feel that permanent changes should only be made once we have proven that the change will achieve the desired effect, and if the patient cannot tolerate weaning from their daytime orthotic.

Appliances—Giving the Joint a Rest

As mentioned in the last chapter, once a diagnosis is made, treatments in our office for TMJ and sleep apnea are very similar, involving orthotics or oral appliances.

With the oral appliance, the condyle and disc are positioned as ideally as possible to stabilize the joint and give it and all the other elements around it time to rest and heal. The goal is for the bones to regenerate, the muscles to relax, the ligaments to heal as much as possible, and for inflammation to be eliminated.

It's similar to treating a broken leg. Once the bone is reset in the correct position, then a cast is applied to hold everything in place for twelve weeks until it heals. Then the cast is removed. The oral appliance is similar to a cast for the jaw.

There are actually two appliances. One appliance is worn during the day when the patient is awake and upright, talking, and even while eating. The daytime appliance fits only on the lower teeth; it is small and compact, allowing for more functionality. The daytime appliance allows the jaw to continue functioning while stabilizing the joint to allow it to heal.

The appliance works because the human body is always remodeling itself. It grows and sheds skin every day. Bones are always changing their shape in response to forces that are applied to them. As long as your heart is beating, you're pumping blood and you're breathing—your body is undergoing changes. It's always trying to get to the most ideal condition that it possibly can, dealing with the forces that are upon it.

If a jaw joint is damaged, particularly to the point where there is bone loss, then supporting it in a normal, stable position can actually allow the bone to start growing back. The bone can start remodeling to create an ideal, functional joint. That healing is completely up to the patient's body—it's the body's choice to try to be as healthy as it can be. The actual changes that occur can be seen in X-rays taken as treatment progresses. On occasion, we've had the opportunity to see images of a joint many years after treatment, and it looks completely different—far more normal—than when the patient first came in.

The second appliance is worn only at night to help control the position of the jaw during sleep—it keeps the condyle and jaw from receding backward and keeps the tongue from falling back into the throat and causing an airway obstruction. The nighttime appliance fits only on the upper teeth and restricts jaw movement a bit more, but it's necessary to protect the TMJ and help prevent airway obstruction.

Together, the two appliances stabilize the joint, keeping the jaw in a protected position for ten to twelve weeks. The only time the appliances are removed is to brush and floss the teeth, or to change out one appliance for the other.

Weaning—the Beginning of the End

After ten to twelve weeks of treatment, which includes multiple office visits (every two weeks) and other integrated treatments (see Chapter 7), the patient is weaned off the daytime appliance.

Weaning begins with reevaluation and imaging—we refer to this as maximum medical improvement (MMI) records. Various medical groups and guidelines have been reviewed to get the consensus that twelve weeks is when the appliance needs to be re-evaluated. So imaging is taken to see what position the jaw joint is in once it has been splinted for three months. The image also looks at how the joint position is affecting the airway, the cervical spine, and other structures.

Photographs are also part of the reevaluation to record the placement of the teeth (which don't change), and to reevaluate the position of the head, neck, and shoulders (posture).

Weaning instructions are then explained to the patient to ensure that they understand the protocol ahead—the daytime appliance is being removed over time, and that leaves the possibility that symptoms will return.

THE ACTUAL WEANING ITSELF IS A FOUR-WEEK PROCESS:

- **Week one:** The daytime appliance is removed for one hour, three times a day—in the morning, afternoon, and just before bedtime. It remains in while eating.

- **Week two:** The appliance is removed two hours at a time, three times a day. It is still left in while eating.

- **Week three:** The appliance is removed three hours at a time, three times a day. The patient still eats with the appliance in. For some patients, this is the last week of treatment with the daytime appliance.

- **Week four:** For those patients who still have the daytime appliance in, it is worn only while eating. After a few days, most patients are entirely off the appliance.

The weaning is structured in such a way because the muscles have the memory of ideal position. They're going to maintain that position for an hour or so. At two hours without the appliance, the muscles are going to start bending to the will of the teeth; wherever the teeth want the muscles to go, they're going to go.

If the teeth are in a place that doesn't agree with the ideal jaw position, which is what happens with most patients, then there will be a discrepancy. But over the course of a month's time, the muscles will very slowly start to adapt.

With the inflammation and pain gone at that point, it's just a matter of having equilibrium—how happy the muscles are versus how much time the teeth are actually meeting. If at night the TM Joints continue to be protected and the muscles are kept happy, then during the day when the patient is awake, the total time that their teeth actually meet is twenty to thirty minutes. When a person is sitting and relaxing—not doing anything—their teeth are actually supposed to be apart. The proper posture is lips together, teeth slightly apart, and the tongue touching the roof of the mouth. The only time teeth come together is during chewing or swallowing. At that point, the teeth close together, the tongue touches the roof of the mouth to push the saliva back down the throat, then the teeth pop apart to the resting position.

> When a person is relaxing, the proper mouth posture is with the lips together, teeth apart, and the tongue touching the roof of the mouth.

The weaning process leverages twenty to thirty minutes of unprotected contact during the day against six to eight hours of protection at night. Usually, patients are able to achieve an equilibrium and they will wean just fine, but some don't have the tolerance and they start sliding back.

During weaning, the patient's symptoms are monitored closely. If their symptoms begin to return, then the weaning failed. For those patients, their body is essentially saying it still likes and needs the support and help of the appliance.

The chief complaint of most patients who struggle with the weaning process is headaches. For ten or more weeks, they've gone without the headaches that plagued them before treatment. Most patients start the weaning process off very positive, very hopeful. Week one, they feel pretty good. Then, in week two, they have a headache. Now, that headache is often completely random—caused by a flu bug or spending too much time at the computer. But they're still hopeful and want to continue with the weaning process, even though in the end, they may be one of the 5 percent that don't successfully wean.

It's crucial for the patient to be honest about their experience during the weaning process. It's human nature, for the most part, to want everything to turn out for the best. But patients are reminded of the importance of being objective. We need to know if everything is functioning better, or worse.

If the weaning process doesn't appear to be working, it can be stopped or slowed. But sometimes a patient is having problems and doesn't report them, and instead goes through the entire weaning process. Then three months later, their headaches have returned and they need treatment again. At that point, Phase I treatment must be done all over again. That can get very expensive.

In our office, only 5 percent of patients do not successfully wean off the appliance the first time.

While 95 percent of patients wean successfully, there are a few exceptions that require a couple of attempts. Some patients, like Laura, have a tougher time of weaning off the daytime appliance. When that happens, the patient typically continues to wear the appliance for another four weeks to ensure long-term stability. Then the weaning process takes place again. We only try that once. If it fails again, we recommend Phase II therapy.

Once the patient is successfully weaned, then only the nighttime appliance is worn long term. It's a little like wearing a brace while playing tennis to keep a bad knee safe.

Some patients are even able to stop wearing the nighttime appliance after a period of time, although that is not recommended. The joint may be corrected, but there is still the potential for additional clenching to occur, creating new damage. What has been happening occasionally is that a successfully weaned TMJ patient will return seven to ten years later with a recurrence of symptoms. We reevaluate for sleep apnea and often find that it has developed over time past the extent that their nighttime TMJ orthotic can help.

Maintenance Care

Similar to going to see your family dentist every six months, patients come back to us for maintenance after they have completed treatment. The length of time between visits varies depending upon the patient's needs. The goal is to ensure their condition remains stable and doesn't worsen, and to ensure their appliance remains in good condition. It is very rewarding to see how the treatment truly changes the lives of the patients we serve.

For that 5 percent of patients who can't or don't wean off the Phase I treatment orthotics, Dr. Ed's side of the practice takes over with Phase II orthodontic treatment. The patient is referred to Dr. Ed, along with information about the current position and stability of the lower jaw and teeth. Armed with that information, he determines what is needed to support the mandible and the relationship between the mandibular condyle and the temporal bone where it will be stable.

CHAPTER 6

Phase II TMJ and Integrative Orthodontic Treatment

rthodontics is about more than straight teeth—it is about functional airways and good health.

At the Centre for Integrative Orthodontics, we use many different tools to achieve optimal results. "Integrative" refers to our use of chiropractic, nutritional, myofunctional, and breathing analysis protocols.

At age eight, Molly was undergoing integrative orthodontics, early treatment to expand her upper and lower arches in order to open a deficient nasal airway both to create room for all her permanent teeth, and to correct an upper jaw deficiency. She had just reached the point in her treatment where the expansion had greatly improved her nasal airway, and we were just initiating the phase of treatment to develop the upper jaw forward. At that point, her father got a job transfer and the family moved to Savannah, Georgia. While there, she underwent conventional orthodontic treatment to "finish her case" —the normal type of treatment that is the shortest and easiest path to straight teeth. Three years later, the family moved back, and she returned to our practice for completion of her case.

Unfortunately, the treatment in Savannah had caused her upper jaw skeletal deficiency to become worse than before she had started treatment with us originally and had also caused severe constriction of her nasal and oropharyngeal airways. She was complaining of fatigue, and her parents commented on her "grumpiness." When she left for Savannah, her upper jaw was about four millimeters deficient in an anterior-posterior (front to back) position. Upon her return, it was almost 10 millimeters deficient. Four is easily correctable, but ten is much more difficult. Her upper jaw was basically collapsed in both dimensions: Laterally (side to side) and from front to back. Her airways were compromised and her facial aesthetics had suffered. Due to her airway constriction, her tongue posture had dropped and she had been forced to breathe through her mouth most of the time. This led to her face getting longer, and now she had to strain her facial muscles just to close her lips together. At that point, she needed completely different treatment than if she had been able to stay under our care in the first place. In fact, most of the treatment she received in Savannah would need to be undone, and it would be very difficult to fully correct some of the severe skeletal issues that now existed.

Molly's case demonstrates how skeletal, airway, and neurologic conditions in kids can be severe, and overall, we're finding that these problems are becoming quite common. Now is the time for orthodontists to screen every patient for these types of issues. That screening, and institution of treatment protocols to address any functional and skeletal issues found, must become the new orthodontic paradigm.

Of course, straightening the teeth is also part of our treatment. Our protocols are orthopedic/orthodontic and functional in nature, to better address the skeletal deficiencies and functional abnormalities by remodeling the orofacial structures and instituting therapies to normalize function. There are many terms being presented currently: dentofacial orthopedics, functional orthodontics, airway centered orthodontics, and myofunctional therapy. We prefer integrative orthodontics, because it often requires the talents of more than one practitioner to achieve the best possible result.

Two Types of Phase II TMJ Orthodontic— A Subsection of Integrative Orthodontics (IO)

Phase II treatments are orthodontic/orthopedic in nature, designed to correct skeletal and functional deficiencies and asymmetries by remodeling the facial structure—as much as possible—in patients who did not have these issues addressed when they were younger. We generally can make significant skeletal changes, even in adults.

In our patients with TMJ problems, there are two types of Phase II treatments.

The first type of Phase II treatment is for TMJ patients who do not successfully wean off of the Phase I appliances. For those patients, Phase II treatment can help stabilize the repositioned jaw to prevent reoccurrence of their symptoms, and as we treat, it will also improve their airway. We have found that this type of Phase II treatment opens the airway by about 40 percent and reduces collapse at night by roughly 37 percent.

Dr. Lynn's Phase I TMJ treatment addresses the jaw joints incredibly well, eliminating inflammation in the jaw joint and sufficiently healing and reforming damaged bone in the jaw joints. The telling part of treatment is weaning. That is when we find out whether the patient's body can tolerate not having the constant support previously provided by their orthotics. Approximately 5 percent of our patients cannot wean off their daytime appliance and will experience a partial/

full return of their symptoms. This might be due to neck issues related to forward head posture, or they may not be able to wean because their airways are woefully deficient (because their jaw structure is deficient in size), and they may still have inflammation in their nasal airway. The problem is often that the nasal airway structure is very narrow because the palate is narrow. Since the roof of the mouth (palate) is the floor of the nose, when the palate is narrow, the nasal airway is forced to be narrow too. When the nasal airway is very narrow, the patient is forced to breathe through their mouth a significant amount of time, or for some patients, all the time. That open mouth posture is what leads to muscular forces that disrupt normal facial growth.

As we stated previously, REM sleep is, neurologically, a parasympathetic state, so the nose is more blocked during REM because of soft tissue vascular engorgement, causing the nasal mucosa to have more volume and take up space where air is supposed to flow. It's not really inflammation, it is just that the tissue enlarges because of the increased blood flow. Someone whose nasal passages are blocked during the day to the point of having to breathe through their mouth will have a bigger problem at night (during REM) when the narrow passages are even more constricted by the enlarged soft tissue. This can lead to snoring, UARS, sleep fragmentation, obstructive apnea, and the many related medical issues.

The second type of "Phase II" treatment is provided when our Phase I TMJ patient is able to successfully wean from their appliances, but they see the value in permanently correcting other structural and functional problems so they can be as healthy as possible, even though their jaw joint pain issues have been satisfactorily resolved.

Our integrative orthodontic approach was developed initially to benefit children. Today, it is rare to see a child's face that has developed fully, the way nature intended. That goes back to the anthropological changes studied by Dr. Weston Price and many others—discussed earlier. These changes are associated with things like the introduction of farming, the introduction of grains, and the widespread distribution of sugar. These occurrences have increased inflammation and contributed to the decreases in the size of the jaw and face we see today. Along with those factors, changes in food texture, mainly associated with softer foods—that is, foods requiring less force/action to chew—have reduced the stimulus for bones to grow to their full genetic potential. It is the action of using the jaws, exercising or straining them, that actually makes the bones grow bigger and denser, and to develop to the dimension that is needed for normal function, allowing a healthier state.

The end result, commonly seen in modern society, is less facial development, nasal airways that are forced to be smaller, narrow and underdeveloped upper jaws, a lower jaw set farther back and rotated down from where nature intended it to be (leading, in some patients, to longer faces), along with other factors that influence how large the pharyngeal (throat) airway is. This predisposes kids to disturbed sleep and sleep apnea. We often see patients who have airways so small that they measure "off the standardized scale" as recorded by our 3-D imaging equipment airway volume program.

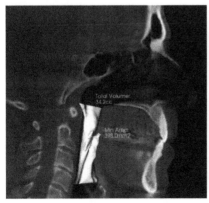 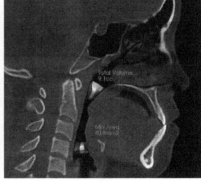

Good airway   Bad airway

We've seen some patients' airways cross-section measured as small as 2 millimeters squared when they're awake! That's like breathing through a coffee stirrer straw. Imagine how bad their airway gets when they are lying down and asleep. Airways almost always have some degree of collapse during sleep. Basically, patients like that are always struggling to survive.

In his studies at Stanford University, professor Christian Guilleminault, MD, a neurologist, discusses the problems with, and solutions for, airway deficiency. A variety of studies show that, especially in children, sleep apnea is a craniofacial structural deficiency (although sometimes obesity can cause sleep apnea in people with a normal facial structure).[26] In order to fix the problem, any craniofacial structural anomalies must be corrected to make the airways as structurally normal as possible. That is what our integrative orthodontic treatment addressed, however, it involves different mechanics and protocols than with normal orthodontic treatment. We make corrections involving maximizing the airway and allowing the patient to breathe through their nose day and night.

We utilize an onsite chiropractic physician to aid diagnosis and treatment, and we refer to osteopaths and other chiropractic physicians in cases that require their help with these cranial deficiencies and distortions.

With integrative orthodontic treatment, the goal is to develop the face to be as symmetrical and completely developed as possible to achieve the most ideal dimensions. Studies show that not only will this lead to better health but faces developed in this manner are also consistently viewed as more attractive. At the beginning of Chapter 1, we shared the anecdote about getting off on the wrong exit and

---

26   Y-S Huang, "Pediatric Obstructive Sleep Apnea and the Critical Role of Oral-Facial Growth: Evidences," *Frontiers in Neurology* 3 (2012): 184.

being unable to find an entry ramp to get back on the highway. That's what it's like for many patients—they've gotten off the road and have gotten farther and farther away from the ideal craniofacial structure.

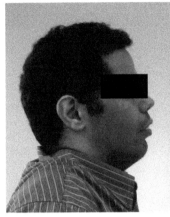 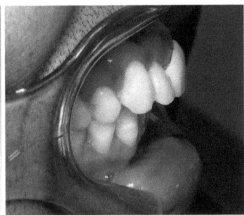

While we have successfully treated seventy-year-old patients whose cranial sutures are not fused, the younger we can start patients with our treatment protocols, the closer to ideal their results will ultimately be.

For instance, if an adult's upper jaw is retruded or set back by 14 millimeters (about a half inch), the integrative orthodontic treatment may only be able to move their upper jaw 9 millimeters forward. (In some cases we can go even further, but in adults this is more difficult and can take more time.) That's such a huge improvement that it usually results in normal tongue posture, corrected function, and an improvement in facial appearance, while also allowing a poorly positioned lower jaw to reposition forward, opening the airway further. The normal tongue posture and function will stabilize the changes in jaw position. That much movement of the upper jaw, along with expansion, can also help open the nasal passages. At some point, forward growth of the upper jaw may be limited in older patients; however, lateral expansion will always provide more room for the tongue and internally broaden the airway—a palate widened correctly will improve the nasal airway.

Changing the structure generally changes the function. Once the facial dimensions are more ideal, then the jaw can function more normally. "Form follows function." In some patients, myofunctional therapy may be necessary to change long standing aberrant muscle functions.

Divine Proportion—The Ideal Face

Determining the ideal facial dimensions is a little like working to achieve divine proportion. As mentioned in Chapter 3, divine proportion is a definition of beauty found everywhere in nature. These proportions promote ideal function, harmony, symmetry, and balance.

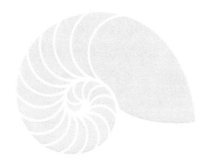

The ancient Greeks discovered that there are certain proportions found in nature, whether in the structure of a snowflake, the way that the stamen and petals on a flower are arranged, or the curve of a nautilus seashell. Everywhere in nature, when things are healthy and functioning ideally, there are certain universal proportions.

Leonardo da Vinci demonstrated the concept of the ideal proportions of the human body with his drawing of the Vitruvian Man, which shows two superimposed male figures within a circle and a square. According to divine proportion, the ideal ratio for parts of the body, including facial components should be 1:1.618. In other words, if the ratio between different areas is close to 1:1.618, then that is considered ideal. For example, if the distance from the top of the head to the bottom of the chin is 1.618, then the side-to-side dimension of the face should be 1. That's a relative ratio. Whatever the numbers are, when everything is ideally balanced for correct function, the proportion should always be 1:1.618.

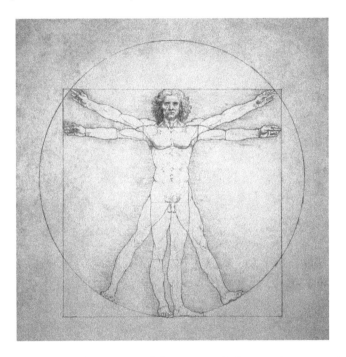

A proportional analysis of the size and shape of a patient's head can help us evaluate how close they are to ideal in order to determine the best mode and direction of desired skeletal changes of treatment. The goal is for everything to be in ideal proportions as much as possible.

Internal variations also help determine treatment. For instance, if someone has a larger tongue, then their arch dimensions should be larger to accommodate the tongue. The teeth are a "cage" for the tongue, so a bigger tongue needs a bigger cage. A size "ten" tongue cannot fit and function correctly inside a size "five" cage.

In addition to the divine proportion providing guidance for treatment, we also look at what it takes to make function normal. Again, a size "five" tongue can't function well inside a size "three" space. Where can it go? Especially if the patient is biting, clenching, and grinding, then the tongue can't go forward without getting bitten by the front teeth. If the tongue doesn't fit its "cage," it generally gets forced back where it blocks the airway. The tongue is taken into consideration when creating a treatment plan; it's crucial to ensure that the structure being created will allow everything to work the way it is supposed to.

Everything must be in proportion. The more symmetrical everything is, the more normal function can become. If one side of the jaw is in proportion but the maladaptive changes reduce the other side, then the spaces that the nerves need to reside in are diminished. If the nerves are trapped because the spaces—even in the bone—are too narrow for them to go through, then nerve pain and inflammation is more likely in those areas. One of the more serious conditions of facial nerve pain is trigeminal neuralgia, involving the three nerve branches which could be experiencing compression in various places. Sometimes it's caused by a structural issue, and if the structural issue is normalized, then the pain can go away.

Reshaping the Face

With traditional orthodontics, the force levels that are used to move teeth are higher than the range where it becomes possible to grow new bone. Traditional orthodontic brackets involve placing a tie around the bracket to firmly hold the wire in place, whether it's an elastic ligature (rubber band-like tie) or a very thin steel wire that is twist-tied over the bracket to lock the wire into place. Those types of brackets and ligatures create a significant force. In traditional orthodontics, the force placed upon the root of the tooth as it is being pushed against the bony wall of the tooth socket is in the range of 80 to 150 grams of force. That amount of force crushes the blood vessels in the socket area, eliminating blood flow to the bone. It also crushes the cells of the periodontal ligament, the fibers that are connected to the roots of the tooth and span the space between the roots and the bone. That causes the bone and other tissues in the area of compression within the socket to die.

The result is an inflammatory response within the bone to clear away all those cells. That creates a void into which the tooth is pushed, and this is considered "normal orthodontic tooth movement." Once the tooth has moved a bit, the pressure decreases a little. Then there is a healing process as the blood supply regenerates. Cells known as osteoclasts and osteoblasts come to repair the damaged area and remodel the socket wall to match the new tooth position. This cycle of destruction and repair happens over and over again, restarted at every orthodontic appointment when the wire is "tightened." The process works as long as teeth are being moved around within existing bone.

> Osteoblast: cell that builds bone
> Osteoclast: cell that removes dead/dying bone

With this type of force, there is no mechanism that allows new bone to grow at the outer surface in the direction that the tooth is being moved. This technique works to move teeth within the already existing bone. If, for example, a tooth is being moved sideways to make the arches wider using these traditional force levels, then the inflammatory response keeps removing the supporting bone. And if the tooth was being moved toward the outer edge of the bone, eventually the tooth would be pushed right out of the bone. This is why doctors using traditional force levels have extreme limitations on dental arch and bone development. If you can't change the dimension of the bone that makes up the part of the jaw in which the teeth are, then you can't treat even moderate dental crowding without extracting teeth.

Obviously, that's a very bad idea, as studies show that space for the tongue is reduced when teeth are extracted. If the skeletal dimension is already too small to allow normal function, it doesn't make sense to use a technique that stands no chance to improve the situation, but certainly has high potential to diminish the skeletal form even further. Orthodontists and general dentists who are practicing traditional orthodontics are limited to moving teeth around within existing bone. Their methods do not allow for the growth of new bone, which is what most patients seem to need.

Also, in the traditional orthodontic paradigm, they believe that palates can only be expanded in younger children (growing individuals) and then only to match the existing lateral (side-to-side) dimension of the lower arch (because they don't have a technique that allows for lateral development of new bone to allow the lower teeth to move to a wider arch form). If the upper and lower teeth already match up laterally, then traditional orthodontists won't use an expander—even if the nasal airway is very narrow—because they think they can't move the lower teeth out wider or they'll push them out of the bone. It's a very limiting philosophy.

Slow and Steady Wins

The integrative orthodontic treatment we provide is based upon the principles of understanding how the cranial bones grow. We have researched and integrated chiropractic, osteopathic, and physiologic principles to create a program that works.

In 1932, researcher A.M. Schwarz found that using significantly lower levels of force could move the tooth within the socket without crushing the blood supply.[27] In 1932, this discovery was purely academic, as no one at that time understood how to achieve that light of a force level on actual patients. This light force level engenders a completely different physiologic mechanism to allow for tooth movement. This technique eliminates the destruction of cells and allows the tooth to move faster. With the higher forces of traditional orthodontics, moving a tooth into position that was formerly occupied by the bony socket takes seven to fourteen days. Using the lower level of force, the teeth move into that position, without inflammation, in about two days.

With the lighter force method, bone has the ability to remodel and grow, since there's no interruption of blood supply. The intact blood supply allows for the immediate activation of osteoclasts, that remove bone physiologically, without an inflammatory response. If a tooth is being moved toward a bony surface using these light forces, osteoclasts remove bone near the tooth, while—through several mechanisms—osteoblastic (bone building) activity is initiated at the surface of the bone. That helps maintain the dimension of the bone in the jaw around the tooth. As the tooth moves toward the surface, new bone is being laid down on the jaw in front of the tooth. As long as the force level is light, the blood supply remains uninterrupted, and there is no inflammatory response in response to cells dying. Then, new bone grows just by having a gentle force activating all the cellular activity. This is similar to bony responses to forces during normal growth.

That's how lower arches can be made wider to accommodate a larger tongue. In fact, when treatment is concluded, imaging frequently shows that there is more bone thickness in the area where new bone was created than there was before the orthodontic treatment

---

27   A. M. Schwarz, "Tissue Changes Incidental to Orthodontic Tooth Movement," *International Journal of Orthodontia and Oral Surgery* 18 (1932): 331.

started. The whole process is basically simulating nature, allowing the skeletal form to become what genetics would have accomplished if functional issues hadn't altered the normal growth.

CASE STUDY: ALEX

Alex presented to Dr. Ed's office while already in the middle of orthodontic treatment at another office. Her treatment had consisted of using traditional (high) force levels. This had resulted in the roots of her anterior teeth being pushed right through the front surface of the bone. There was literally no bone around the roots of those teeth for their entire front surface, as shown on the following upper skull image and on the X-ray image. Alex was told that these teeth needed to be extracted. She came to our office with the hope that her teeth could somehow be saved. At the age of fourteen, Alex faced the real possibility of losing all of her upper front teeth.

Dr. Ed, after evaluating the situation, told Alex that he'd do his best to regrow bone for her, and that he had been successful with other patients presenting with similar issues. Alex's braces were changed so the light forces needed could be employed. By using the techniques and principles of tooth movement described previously, Dr. Ed was able to reposition Alex's anterior teeth, growing new bone in front of the roots of all those teeth, as shown in the following images, thus saving those teeth.

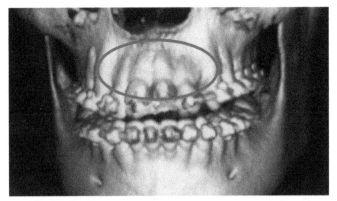

Before treatment: upper anterior teeth pushed out of the bone.

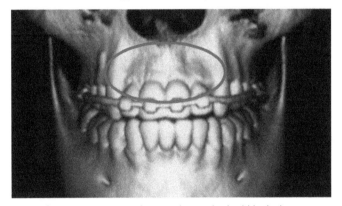

After treatment: upper front teeth roots back within the bone.

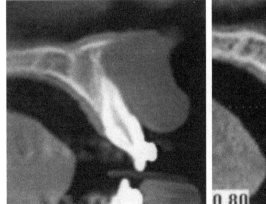
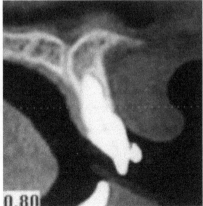

Before treatment   After treatment

Despite our ability to make skeletal changes even in adults, it's always best to treat as early as possible, especially with certain problems, such as those involving the lower anterior teeth. Since it's difficult to grow bone forward in the area around the lower front teeth because the roots are narrow and therefore less effective at stimulating new bone growth, typically only about a millimeter or two of forward bony growth can be accomplished in this region. This may be a limiting factor in treatment. Fortunately, we can change the position of the entire lower jaw to reposition it forward for patients who have receded lower jaws.

There are certain cases where the lower jaw grows to a normal dimension, but the lower front teeth are set back, resulting in a big discrepancy. That can happen when the front teeth have a significant vertical overlap when biting the back teeth together. That becomes a dilemma to fix when facial growth is finished—for girls around age fourteen or fifteen, and for boys around age seventeen. There are skeletal evaluations we can make, looking at cervical vertebrae, to determine if there's any facial growth remaining. When that discrepancy arises in a young child, corrective treatment can make everything grow normally from that point on. If the problem isn't corrected until the teen years or later, it may be too late to get a full correction, and functional and aesthetic compromises may need to be made. Again, depending on the issues, timing is essential to make the structures as ideal as possible.

Integrative orthodontic treatment for people who have completed their growth can still be successful. The amount of bony changes possible may be more limited. One limiting factor is time. Sometimes corrections toward the ideal may be very large. We are currently treating an adult patient who came to our office with a 28-millimeter skeletal discrepancy between the alignment of the upper and lower jaws. His lower jaw and chin were very prominent. The patient didn't want the surgical correction that could have corrected this discrepancy completely. Without surgery, it isn't possible to make his lower jaw less prominent. We certainly can develop his small upper jaw forward. At the time of this writing, his upper jaw is around 9 millimeters forward of its starting dimension and significantly expanded, and we will be able to improve that dimension further. He already looks much better than his initial appearance and there have been huge improvements in his ability to breathe normally and sleep well. The corrections won't leave him with ideal proportions, but his dental bite will be corrected, and his functional issues and appearance will be greatly enhanced.

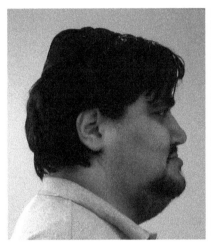 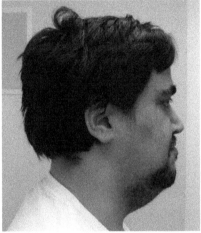

Before treatment   Mid-treatment, 30 months

Another issue is long-standing aberrant muscle pressure. For example, trying to move teeth forward for someone who has overly tense lips may be limiting—at some point, their lips may apply enough pressure to inhibit new growth. This is why we utilize myofunctional therapy in our practice. It normalizes muscle function, allowing better outcomes.

In fact, when we simply use brackets and light orthodontic forces on teeth, the maximum forward movement seems to be about 5 millimeters. In most other practices, that's considered a significant discrepancy, and is either referred for surgical correction or left unaddressed. When greater correction is needed, we use additional techniques.

Dr. Ed has developed other techniques that allow for more forward movement. These are more dentofacial orthopedics than orthodontics and may involve an appliance that effectively brings forward the entire upper jaw (reverse-pull face mask). With this treatment, the teeth are anchored with a dental appliance in order to translate the force to the bone. That allows the entire maxilla (upper jaw) to move forward, a complicated movement because it connects to eight other bones, and the sutures (seams) between all those bones are remodeling. When the treatment is complete, patients often look very different. For instance, it's not uncommon for a person to have developed more prominent cheekbones once the treatment is complete. Because we are correcting deficiencies and treating toward divine proportion, patients look better and function better, and corrections are more stable.

This type of treatment takes anywhere from four months to two or more years, depending on the patient's need. Expansion and leveling and/or aligning teeth typically takes less time, while moving the maxilla (upper jaw) can take eight or nine months. Vertical changes such as stimulating amounts like five millimeters of vertical bone growth while moving lower teeth, can make the entire treatment time take two or more years.

Dentofacial Appliances

There are several appliance options available for use in dentofacial orthopedics. Some have been around for quite a while, while others are new to the scene.

For example, if the goal is to move the upper jaw forward only around 5 millimeters, then the Damon System for braces will do the job.

If the x-ray and CBCT (cone beam computed tomography) images show that the airway is very deficient, that deficiency is because the palatine bone (behind the maxilla) is too far back. Growing the front of the maxillary bone forward won't change that back position. Instead, what's needed is an appliance to bring the entire upper jaw (maxillary-palatine complex) forward. This would be a situation that calls for a reverse-pull face mask.

Traction appliances have been used for years for patients that have a prominent lower jaw. Traction involves moving and remodeling the bones and the sutures (or seams) of the cranium. Most dentists are taught that all the sutures fuse together during the teenage years, however, the medical literature shows that is not true. In adults, the sutures between bones get more complex and more intricate (think overlapping and interlocking), and moving them initially is a very conservative, gentle, and slow process of remodeling. At times, the bone from one side of a suture may be so extended within the suture that it locks around bone from the other side. Since traction would involve pushing bone against bone, the initial part of this treatment requires osteoclastic and osteoblastic (bone-building) activity. Those locked bones have interferences that can be moved at roughly an eighth of a millimeter per week. This initially requires osteoclastic activity to take away bone that is interlocked and engages with light pressure when movement is started. Once the interferences are removed through remodeling, then the bone can be moved at the same rate as in a child. For a midpalatal suture and palatal expansion, that rate is about a half a millimeter per week. For reverse-pull traction, it is more about force levels, which can be the same as for a child after about six weeks of light traction.

Whenever there is an inflammatory response, we use cold laser treatment to keep it in check. That's just one of the integrated therapies offered (see Chapter 7).

There are several appliances used in our treatment regimen, including expanders (Schwartz, SlimLine Hyrax, Quadhelix, ALF, and Bent Wire System), Damon System for braces, and Myobrace®. We do not receive money from these companies or individuals, these appliances just consistently have worked well.

Expanders—Same Tool, Different Technique

Expanders are a broad category of appliance that exerts force on the palate to push it laterally and sometimes anteriorly. There are many styles of expanders, and they all work essentially the same way: by applying force to make skeletal and dental changes. Traditional orthodontics use expanders to apply great force to push the palate laterally. Because of the force levels and the inflammatory response at the bony socket, most doctors believe that they must tear the mid-palatal suture apart before the teeth are pushed out of the bone. Light force expanders work with the body's physiological mechanisms to create new bone. ALF appliances are a type of light force "expansion" appliance with a great potential to move cranial bones. We use it in our office along with a cranial chiropractor to check these patients and make any adjustments needed with lighter force.

Here again, we use a lighter force. The sutures allow the bones to independently have some slight movement, which helps in a lot of different ways. Imagine, for example, getting whacked on the side of the head. Because the sutures have some independent movement, they act as shock absorbers and protect the bones from fracture. There's also a flow of cerebral spinal fluid that works its way up and down the spinal cord and circulates around the brain. Cerebral spinal fluid is a circulatory system that brings nutrients to these structures and removes waste and toxins from these areas. It is the movement of the cranial bones which makes it circulate the way it's supposed to.

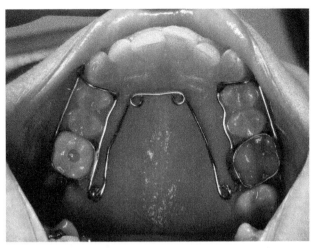
Palatal expander using light force.

Proper expansion using less force, which makes the nasal airway wider, allows for bone growth in the mid-palatal suture, or the seam in the roof of the mouth. In order for the upper jaw bones to move apart, new bone must grow to fill the void in the middle where the two parts are pushed apart laterally. The fibers that run between the two bones stimulate osteoblast activity when they're stretched. So, new bone grows to fill in the places where the bones have moved apart. The bones should not be moved apart any faster than new bones can fill in. The expansion rate that seems to allow this is about a half of a millimeter per week.

Unfortunately, when traditional orthodontists use rapid palatal expansion to tear the suture apart, healing of the wound created when the suture tears frequently leads to regions of bony fusion across the palate. These areas of fusion make the palate function as one bone, which significantly restricts its ability to flex and move normally. As the maxilla has connections to eight other bones, this likely has a negative impact on their ability to move as much as is ideal. That happens when orthodontists believe they must use high, rapid force to tear open the suture. When they use rapid palatal expansion, they also generally only expand enough to match the dimension of the lower arch. Instead of expanding to the 10 or 12 millimeters the patient actually needs to get normal function and open up the nasal airway, they expand 4 millimeters because that's what makes the upper teeth line up correctly with the lower teeth. They don't believe they can widen the lower dental arch. When expansion is enough to allow for normal function, it has the best chance at being stable. Ten to 12 millimeters of expansion is likely to be more stable than 4 millimeters if the arch dimension at 4 millimeters doesn't improve the nasal airway adequately and doesn't allow the tongue to posture up in the palate (where it belongs most of the time) comfortably.

But studies actually show that even at age seventy, the cranial suture is still viable and expandable—if it hasn't been fused by rapid palatal expansion or some other pathological traumatic event.[28] When the suture is torn apart, it heals with bony fusions. Using light forces, the dental arch can be made wider, because bone can be grown in the direction of the movement of teeth. This can allow for enough room for the tongue, but the nasal airway can't be improved through expansion in these circumstances. For patients with bony fusion at the midpalatal suture, surgery by an otolaryngologist (ENT physician) is the only solution. This is why one of the questions we ask people is if they have had previous orthodontics or expansion.

Our oldest expansion patient to date is seventy-two years old (actually there are two such patients).

We had a forty-seven-year-old periodontist who began treatment with Dr. Lynn for chronic migraines, and neck and back pain. He successfully completed his Phase I TMJ treatment but could not wean. He had a lower tooth that had been totally blocked out of his arch, was

---

28   Bernal Revlo and Leonard S. Fishman, "Maturational evaluation of ossification of the midpalatal suture," AJODO 105, no. 3 (March 1994): 288–292, https://doi.org/10.1016/S0889-5406(94)70123-7.

diagnosed with sleep apnea, and was considering rhinoplasty because he did not like the appearance of his nose. To make a long story short, Dr. Ed was able to address his dental issues, create a balanced face by aligning all his teeth without extraction (which made his nose look smaller), and improve his airway so a follow up home sleep test showed a normal AHI.

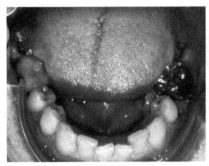 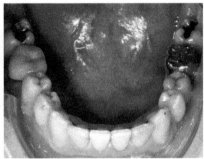

Before treatment   After treatment

Damon Braces—Passive Ligation System

The Damon Braces System is what allows us to use the light forces in treatment. With Damon braces, there are no ties to hold the wire in place. Damon braces use what's known as *passive ligation*, which means the wire is not tied tightly to the bracket, and the force levels used to move the teeth are light in comparison to the usual orthodontic force levels at about 20 percent of the usual force.

Please understand, a bonded orthodontic bracket is simply a handle by which we can "grab" the tooth to move it. It is important that we don't grab it too hard!

Damon braces are composed of brackets that adhere to the teeth, similar to traditional braces, but the difference is in the wire and the way it engages the brackets. Instead of the ties, the brackets have "gates" that close to hold the wire in place. However, the wire itself is "freewheeling" within the bracket. It has the ability to move back and forth within the bracket as it rebounds gently, trying to return to its "straight" form, taking the teeth along for the ride. The wires used early in treatment with Damon brackets are light in the force levels they exert. It is with these light early wires that new bone can be developed.

Myobrace—A Physiological Treatment

Myobrace is a soft, flexible appliance that looks like an athletic mouth guard but is actually a highly engineered, three-stage appliance system designed to correct problems with upper and lower jaw development. The technology was developed in 1981 by Dr. Chris Farrell of Australia.

Myobrace at a young age is ideal for opening the nasal airway, making it easier to breathe correctly. It also promotes normal function by slightly nudging the teeth out wider, and it helps correct tongue posture by retraining the tongue to be up in the roof of the mouth. The tongue functioning properly and positioned in the palate most of the time, along with nasal breathing, is nature's palatal expander.

Myofunctional exercises accompany treatment with Myobrace. This is an essential aspect of treatment that results in successful outcomes. There are other systems available that do not integrate an exercise program. These alternative treatment modalities may seem similar, but they are not as effective and take a lot longer. These exercises, or activities, are basically physical therapy for the facial muscles and the tongue, and they vary depending on patients' needs. Patients are granted access to the activities through the Myobrace company website, and as a certified provider, we get a record of when patients log on. This helps us track whether they're going to the site to do their exercises. Obviously, successful treatment is dependent upon patient cooperation.

The purpose of the Myobrace and the accompanying exercises is to normalize function at a point in time when the structural discrepancies haven't resulted in large developmental problems. The tongue is supposed to reside in the roof of the mouth, touching "the spot" (the soft tissue behind the front teeth), about 85 percent of the time. When the tongue is up there, it's stimulating both lateral and forward growth of the upper jaw. The pressure of the tongue is thought to help stimulate CSF circulation along with other physiological benefits.

Frankly, as stated above, the best expander on the planet is the tongue. When the tongue and facial muscles function normally in the early stages of life, everything grows the way it's supposed to. That's how Myobrace works. It nudges things in a direction that improves function and promotes the normal development of structures.

Once a patient gets used to wearing the appliance and can wear it through the night, they only have to wear it one hour in the evening along with sleeping with the appliance in. In the one waking hour when they're wearing it, they have to keep their lips together, keep their tongue up in the roof of their mouth, and breathe through their nose.

When used as part of a comprehensive program to make function more normal, Myobrace and myofunctional therapy help stabilize other treatments. These are just two of the integrative treatments we use to help patients.

CHAPTER 7
Integrative Treatments

Whenen Jamison came in for an evaluation, he had pain all over his body. His physical issues were so significant that his brain had put him in a sympathetic (fight-or-flight) state, causing his body to make multiple postural compensations to keep his airway open and keep everything working as well as his compromised structure could manage. One shoulder was higher than the other, his hips were canted (causing him balance issues), and his neck was significantly out of alignment. He had been diagnosed with scoliosis. Again, the brain will choose straining body parts and pain over loss of function in what it considers critical areas, and it considers breathing to be the most critical function that must be maintained.

By the time he came to us for a consultation, he was working a job from home that required minimal effort and, other than doctor's appointments, rarely left the house. He was just getting by and ultimately would need a lot of "unraveling" to get him back to functioning normally.

The comprehensive evaluation and review of his health history revealed that his entire upper jaw was displaced to the left about five millimeters, and the right side of his face appeared to be compressed in. Interestingly, photos of him years before, prior to wearing braces, showed that his jaw had better orientation at that time. It became clear that his jaw was in a better position before he underwent orthodontic treatment to correct his "crooked teeth."

We determined that his "primary injury" actually alternated between his neck and lower back. The reason for those primary injuries turned out to be an obstructed nasal and oropharyngeal airway. His brain was forcing postural changes to keep his airway open, but it was possible that he also had actual damage either to the neck or lower back—or even both—that was causing his body to compensate. So, he had several issues that needed to be addressed—any one, or any combination of which could have been causing his body to go into a sympathetic state. We utilized other health professionals to work in tandem with us while we addressed his airway issues.

Jamison's first stage of treatment addressed structural changes to take stress off his neck. He also received treatment from a chiropractic physician specializing in cranial adjustments, who worked on unlocking Jamison's cranial sutures. A special intraoral appliance helped take pressure off the sutures and allow cranial movement to become balanced and regular (ALF). This would allow cerebral spinal fluid flow to return to normal, which typically would help alleviate his head pain.

He also went to one of our "in-house" partner providers, a chiropractor, who addressed his lower back issues. At the time of this writing, he was also beginning to consider treatment by an ENT for his deviated septum, although the palatal expansion we were starting—in conjunction with a traction appliance to bring his rotated maxilla forward and to the right—should improve his poor nasal airway.

Addressing the Primary in Order

Jamison's case demonstrates the need for an integrated treatment plan to resolve the multiple issues that most patients face. This comprehensive treatment often requires care by both in-house and partner health care providers.

Based upon our neurological evaluations, we're often able to identify the primary problem that the patient needs treated first, in accordance with the hierarchy of what the brain prioritizes. Then, depending on what the primary injury is, we either initiate treatment or begin working with other providers to address each issue in the correct sequence.

For example, if a patient's jaw is clearly out of alignment, then most likely there's some damage happening in the TMJ. But that damage may be the result of a problem somewhere else—maybe in their lower back, their knee, their foot, or elsewhere. Every time, for example, their foot hurts or is strained enough to alarm the brain, they clench their teeth, smashing their condyle into the base of their skull, causing damage. If the evaluation determines that the primary structure is outside the license of what we can do in our offices, then the patient must be referred elsewhere for their initial treatment. They may need to first see a chiropractor, an ENT, a neurologist, a podiatrist, or whomever else is appropriate to treat their primary issue, before coming back to us to get treatment for their jaw, if it is still needed. To do otherwise is treating the primary out of sequence, and that will never result in the healing the patient needs. These non-TMJ patients present to our office about 10–15 percent of the time. We have many "partner" doctors who like treating the patients we refer to them because "they all get better."

Dr. Steven Olmos, whose protocol we follow in treating these craniofacial pain/TMJ patients, says that addressing problems out of order is "shimming" away from what the brain considers the worst issue and has opted to protect. Think of wearing a cast on a healthy leg. If their other leg actually needs the cast, placing the cast on the wrong (healthy) leg may actually put even more load and strain on the leg that actually should have been treated. Addressing structures in the incorrect sequence can actually make the patient worse and cause new strains and stresses.

For instance, let's say a patient complains of jaw pain and the doctor creates an oral splint that changes the jaw posture as a way to heal what is diagnosed as TMJ. However, the jaw pain is only being caused by compensations the body is making because of the brain's drive to protect a lower back injury. That splint, then, is not allowing the TMJ to heal, and is creating another situation for the brain to have to adjust for. That can force the body to compensate even more, possibly in previously unaffected areas—all while a primary lower back injury remains untreated. If the compensations are more strenuous and the patient continues clenching, pain levels can actually increase from this (out of sequence) treatment.

That is why it's critical to really figure out what's primary and address things in the correct order. It is also why the patient may require treatment from multiple providers. But that treatment must be coordinated so that each structural issue is addressed in the proper sequence.

Unfortunately, what often happens is that providers immediately want to address all of the problems that fall within the scope of their license, without understanding the need to address what is the primary issue in the correct order.

As another illustration of this, let's say two patients have almost identical pain symptoms in the jaw area. They go to the same dentist, one who is trained to treat TMJ with splint therapy. The dentist evaluates the jaw on each patient and finds that they are sore and tender to the touch. Both patients receive splint therapy. The problem is that one patient is TMJ primary; and for that patient, the splint therapy is appropriate and successful. For the other patient, however, the TMJ is not primary—it may be that their lower back is actually causing their secondary jaw joint pain. The splint therapy makes their condition worse. The splint actually puts more stress and strain into the symptomatic TMJ area because now it is fighting against part of the compensation that the brain has figured out. The dentist is then confused about one case resolving successfully and the other not. And that unresolved patient is still in pain and unhappy. The patient, and even the dentist, may then say, "This TMJ stuff doesn't work."

That's what happened to Jamison. His problem was initially an airway issue. But when the problem was identified by an orthodontist as being an "open bite" and braces were then used to close that bite, Jamison actually ended up in worse shape than before treatment—the braces made his airway worse. Since the obstruction in his nose was the primary problem, his tongue protruded between his front teeth in an effort to open his airway. When the orthodontist closed down his open bite without making sure he could breathe through his nose, it actually made it even harder for him to breathe. It reduced space for his tongue and caused his lower jaw to move backward to further close his airway (and his nose still did not work). His brain and body then began creating new structural compensations to allow him to breathe—to survive. That ended up causing him years of unnecessary pain.

Yes, his teeth looked straight after he wore braces. But they were straightened in a boney base that was already underdeveloped (at age fourteen). Over time, as he continued to grow, that discrepancy became even greater and his dental malocclusion returned. Twenty years earlier, when his jaw development was less compromised, it would have been much easier to fix that discrepancy. By the time he sought treatment with us, it had become an extremely difficult correction.

By unlocking his cranial sutures, we began developing everything to a more balanced condition, and ultimately changed the position and skeletal shape of his jaw and moved his teeth to a more ideal alignment. Without making sure that he had a functioning nasal airway, the corrections made would not have been stable.

Adjunctive Treatments

According to guidelines published by the United States surgeon general (David Satcher) in 2000, dentists are licensed to diagnose and treat dental and structural maladies of the head and neck that are related to craniofacial pain.[29] The dental licenses that we hold allow us to treat patients using a number of innovative therapies. Here are some of the latest treatments that we're using as of 2018.

COLD LASER

"Cold laser" therapy is used on almost every patient because it does so many good things that are necessary for treatment. The term "cold laser" refers to the fact it will not cut or burn tissue. It is also referred to as low-level laser therapy, high-intensity laser therapy, or photobio-modulation therapy (PBMT). We use the Multiwave Locked System (MLS) Therapy Laser, which is the only laser that utilizes dual wavelengths of light. Studies show that syncing the two wavelengths of light maximizes healing and also has the effect of reducing inflammation and pain.[30] It also utilizes a third wavelength of light (infrared) to

---

29   Department of Health and Human Services, "2000 Surgeon General's Report on Oral Health in America," National Institute of Dental and Craniofacial Research, July 2000, https://www.nidcr.nih.gov/research/data-statistics/surgeon-general.

30   Anna Kuryliszyn-Moskal et al., "The influence of Multiwave Locked System (MLS) laser therapy on clinical features, microcirculatory abnormalities and selected modulators of angiogenesis in patients with Raynaud's phenomenon," *Clin Rheumatol.* 34, no. 3 (May 2014): 489–496, https://doi.org/10.1007/s10067-014-2637-8.

increase blood flow to the injured area which aids healing.

Cold laser can also be used for diagnosis, which helps target therapy. Dentists can actually use the cold laser anywhere on the body (except the eyes), as long as it is for diagnostic purposes. But only in the areas within the scope of dentistry can they use a cold laser for treatment. It's similar to taking a patient's pulse using their wrist or taking their blood pressure using a cuff—these are methods for measuring general health which is directly related to what we do. Similarly, a dentist can prescribe a blood test and have a full panel done because the patient's overall health affects their treatment. Then, based on the findings of all the tests, the patient may be referred to a complementary health provider for treatment. While we may be able to use cold laser therapy on someone's foot, for diagnosis, it is outside the scope of our license to use it for treatment. So, we refer the patients we suspect of having foot issues to a podiatrist, a chiropractor, an orthopedic surgeon, or whomever seems most appropriate for treatment.

In addition to diagnosis, cold laser offers a number of benefits in treatment. These include reducing pain, reducing inflammation, accelerating the rate of orthodontic tooth movement, and increasing the speed of healing.

Since inflammation reduces blood flow, by using cold laser therapy to reduce the body's inflammatory response, treatment goes faster. Studies have shown that laser therapy can reduce inflammation and swelling in an affected area.[31] It's such a significant reduction of inflammation and pain that after application of a laser treatment, the brain no longer considers an affected area as being primary. Neurologic testing a patient for the sympathetic state before and after cold laser therapy helps us determine the primary site. If the source of the

---

31   Morena Petrini et al., "Effect of pre-operatory low-level laser therapy on pain, swelling, and trismus associated with third-molar surgery," *Med Oral Patol Oral Cir Bucal* 22, no. 4 (June 2017): e467–e472, https://doi.org/10.4317/medoral.21398.

issue that is causing the problem isn't also addressed, the laser treated site will usually return to its pretreatment condition. When the source is also addressed, laser treatment will lead to faster healing and less residual pain during treatment.

Laser therapy also helps bones remodel faster, which helps teeth move faster. [32] Studies in orthodontics show that if teeth are extracted and then other teeth are being slid into the space, using cold laser therapy can make that movement happen in about two-thirds the time it would normally take. [33] Cold laser therapy also makes the movement of teeth less painful, whether or not an extraction is involved. Using cold laser after "tightening" braces can leave the patient with less pain and aid in faster movement of the teeth.

Cold laser treatments also noticeably reduce pain. One of our orthodontic patients was running late to a meeting one day, so he decided to forgo his cold laser therapy at his appointment. He returned later for laser treatment that same day because he realized, while in his meeting, that he was far less comfortable without having had the laser therapy we usually provide.

For many patients, the pain relief from cold laser treatment is immediate. For some, the pain relief takes a little longer—maybe twenty to forty minutes. On occasion, a patient may need more than one treatment to relieve pain—that's because there are many drivers of inflammation. For instance, if someone sprains an ankle, they'll have an inflammatory cascade. Even though inflammation may be reduced in one area, it's building at the same time in other areas. So, multiple

---

32 M. V. da Silva Sousa et al., "Influence of Low-Level Laser on the Speed of Orthodontic Movement," *Photomed Laser Surg.*, Jan 23, 2011 {epubl ahead of print}.

33 M. Youssef, S. Ahkar, E. Hamade, N. Gutknecht, F. Lampert, and M. Mir, "The Effect of Low-Level Laser Therapy During Orthodontic Movement: A Preliminary Study," *Laser Med Sci.* 23, no. 1, (Jan 2008): 27–33; G. Doshi-Mehta and W. A. Bhad-Pati, "Efficacy of Low-Intensity Laser Theraphy in Reducing Treatment Tie and Orthodontic Pain: A Clinical Investigation," *Am J Orthod Dentofacial Orthop* 141, no. 3 (March 2012): 289–97.

laser treatments may be needed to get the full effect. Our patients receive doctor directed therapy every 2/4/7/14/30 days depending upon their situation. Orthodontic patients are lasered, at a minimum, at every regular orthodontic appointment.

Cold laser also works on trigger points.[34] Traditionally, trigger points have been addressed by using a syringe to inject an anesthetic into the joint to alleviate some pressure build up. Cold laser achieves the same effect without using a needle—great news since most people aren't fond of needles.

Trigger points are fairly easy to find. John F. Kennedy's personal physician, Janet Travell, wrote a two-volume textbook mapping them out, and charts are available that differentiate them all. We also find trigger points during our detailed head-and-neck cranial exam on patients when looking for areas that are tender or painful. There is approximately an 80 percent agreement if you overlay a map of trigger points and acupuncture points.

Trigger points often refer pain to another area of the body. For instance, the sternocleidomastoid, which is a muscle that runs down both sides and the front of the neck, refers pain to a number of the teeth. It's somewhat common for people to mistakenly believe they've got a toothache when they're actually experiencing pain because of the sternocleidomastoid muscle and the body's neuropathways. When a patient identifies one tooth that is the source of the pain, other teeth around it may also appear sensitive. But a toothache usually involves only one tooth. If cold laser application to the sternocleido-mastoid muscle makes the dental pain go away, then the tooth wasn't a problem, and it was more likely pain referred by neuropathways. We test this by applying pressure to the trigger point; if that results in pain

---

34 Trigger points are hyperirritable spots in the fascia which surrounds skeletal muscle. There are palpable nodes and pressure can often elicit local or referred pain. Frequently they can feel like tender knots in a muscle that people try to massage away.

in the tooth, then we know the trigger point is the cause.

Unfortunately, we've seen patients who have had a tooth extracted, but that extraction didn't relieve their pain. How frustrating! That's a pretty good indicator that the sternocleidomastoid may have been the cause of the pain—and the tooth may not have needed extraction.

Cold laser also decreases healing time and can minimize scarring in trauma patients. We've used it on patients who have suffered facial trauma from a car accident or from a sports injury. Sometimes, they are sent in by a plastic surgeon who has helped them with reconstruction, but there is still a dental aspect to their injuries. Cold laser promotes increased cellular activity and reduces inflammation, helping reduce the instance of fibrous tissue that results in scarring. For instance, one of our patients, a teenaged male, was accidentally hit in the face by a baseball bat during a game. He came into our office straight from the hospital after the plastic surgeon sewed him back together and he received intensive laser therapy daily. Four days after his initial cold laser therapy in our office, his plastic surgeon commented that he looked like he had been healing for two weeks.

Cold laser helps reduce Phase I TMJ treatment from six months to as little as twelve weeks. Getting the ligaments that support the jaw to heal can take a long time (six to nine months). Without cold laser, the therapy can take a year or longer.

ELECTRO THERAPEUTIC POINT STIMULATION (ETPS)

Part of the theory in Chinese medicine is that there is chi (Qi), or energy, flowing through the body. That chi can be blocked at certain points. When it's blocked, it can cause pain, disease, and illness. Acupuncture opens up those points and allows the chi to flow correctly.

One way to open up those points without using acupuncture needles is with Electro Therapeutic Point Stimulation (ETPS). ETPS applies a small electrical current to what are known as acupuncture *distant points*. A distant point is a point that, when stimulated, affects a distant body part. While there are a number of distant points on the body, as dentists, we treat the points that are in the hands, which are beneficial to the face and jaw. ETPS is slightly more effective than laser treatment for addressing acupressure points and is used on people who are more comfortable with alternative medicine. The beauty of the technology is that it emits a tone when the distant point is located, making its application very accurate.

ACUPRESSURE

Another treatment derived from Chinese medicine for unblocking chi is acupressure. Acupressure is basically applying pressure to the body's acupressure or trigger points to help the muscles relax. The great thing about acupressure is that the patient can be taught how to do it to themselves.

INJECTIONS

Injections are a last line of defense in our offices for a patient who has pain for which other treatments are not as effective. For instance, an injection of just a little bit of lidocaine every six to nine months provided pain relief for one of our patients. Today, he is stable enough to have them only every two or three years. For him, it was just a matter of breaking the cycle of pain. For some people, a single injection will do the trick. With all the other tools we have in our arsenal, we can usually achieve relief for patients without injections. We refer patients who need prolo therapy (an injection technique used to heal damaged ligaments) to other talented practitioners in our area who specialize in this treatment.

CHIROPRACTIC

When our patients' issues involve the jaw or areas of the head and neck, our in-office chiropractor, Dr. Wells, can perform therapy to the appropriate associated areas. This helps ensure that the treatment doesn't further complicate a trapped or nonmoving maxilla or skull. It also aids to make our treatments more effective. Dr. Wells also directs myofunctional therapy, which is covered in-depth in the next chapter.

NUTRITIONAL SUPPLEMENTS

Nutritional supplement recommendations for every patient include a good multivitamin, and vitamins B, C, and D. We also recommend that every patient increases their magnesium intake. Magnesium is found in the nerve junction and essentially turns off the pain impulse. Chronic pain patients have depleted the magnesium in the nerve junction; that's why they can't turn off the pain. Magnesium is also a muscle relaxant that helps a person sleep. It can take several months to restore the magnesium in the body.

HOMEOPATHIC NASAL SPRAYS

Many of our patients also benefit from using Xlear Nasal Spray, an over-the-counter, drug-free option that is made of saline, grapeseed extract, and xylitol. Spraying with Xlear at bedtime helps deflame the nasal passages to improve nasal breathing and relieve snoring for many patients. Patients who don't get relief with Xlear are moved on to True Functional nasal spray, one of the more recent entries into the market.

Other Providers

When the patient's primary turns out to be something outside the realm of our license, we have established relationships with other providers who we refer our patients to. We communicate our findings about the patient with these providers to help them effectively target their treatment, but they conduct their own exams to confirm our findings before determining what treatment to use. Then, as the primary injuries dictate, patients are sent back to us for those treatments that are within our scope.

That chain of referral providers is part of our integrated team approach. When patients need care from outside providers, we act as the "quarterback" to help guide treatment and determine what comes next as each primary is revealed.

We work with providers who understand the primary injury concept. That's especially difficult for chiropractors who are taught that the world revolves around the first cervical vertebrae or the pelvis. Instead of addressing the actual site of the injury, which may be somewhere else in the spine, those teachings center on the idea that, for instance, by ensuring the first cervical vertebrae is positioned correctly, all of a patient's issues can be resolved. But the first cervical vertebrae may at some point have to make some compensatory changes to accommodate that other damage. Without fixing the damaged area, the first cervical vertebrae will keep being a problem because the brain and body must maintain a certain amount of balance. Once that original problem is corrected, then anything else out of place will move back into position on its own since the displacements only occurred to relieve the strain caused by the original displaced vertebrate.

Once we explain the concept of addressing the primary injury to other providers, then some of them—chiropractors in particular—actually find it so useful that they start evaluating their patients the same way.

Here are some of the other providers we work with outside the practice.

EAR, NOSE, AND THROAT SPECIALIST (ENT)

For many patients who have already undergone high-force rapid palatal expansion and now have a fused palate—their left and right cranial bones are no longer separate—we can still make their upper jaw dimension bigger by using low forces. But nothing can be changed down the midline, meaning their nasal airway cannot be improved with the treatment we offer. Improving the nasal airway is critical to their treatment, but at that point, it becomes a surgical procedure that must be performed by an ENT. We also commonly refer patients to an ENT when we find inflamed tonsils and adenoids, a deviated septum, concha bullosa, and swelling bodies.

SLEEP PHYSICIANS, NEUROLOGISTS, AND PULMONOLOGISTS

When a patient is suspected of having sleep apnea, they are referred for a sleep study. A board-certified sleep physician reviews our request and provides a diagnosis once the study is completed. Although the orthodontic and TMJ treatments we offer may inadvertently help patients with sleep apnea, a proper diagnosis is imperative. The results of the study must be read and diagnosed by a sleep physician.

The results of the study may reveal the need for other providers. For instance, some patients have sleep disorders that are not sleep apnea. Neurologic sleep disorders require special referrals. Restless leg syndrome is one such disorder, and we have found that sometimes, it is something we can affect positively.

Other conditions such as circadian rhythm disorders or narcolepsy may require the help of a neurologist. Patients with pulmonary disease are referred to pulmonologists.

PODIATRIST

Patients with foot disorders are generally referred to a foot doctor.

That condition may be an inflamed peroneal nerve in the foot or maybe Morton's neuroma, either of which may be affecting their posture or making them clench their teeth. The podiatrist's solutions may include foot orthotics or even surgery.

CHIROPRACTORS

We look to chiropractic providers outside of our practice when the issues involve other areas of the body that can be helped by spinal adjustments. We have NUCCA, SOT, and Activator specialists to help our patients with their varied needs.

ORTHOPEDISTS, SURGEONS, AND ORAL SURGEONS

Referral to an orthopedist is indicated in fewer than 2 percent of cases, with typically only the most severe requiring some sort of surgical correction. For instance, one patient had condyle erosion that was so severe she needed a condylar replacement. She was seventeen years old at the time of her surgery and we, post surgically, had to make a nighttime appliance to prevent her lower jaw from falling back to block her airway.

PEDIATRIC PROVIDERS

Ehlers-Danlos syndrome is a genetic connective tissue disorder where all the joints are hypermobile: the spine, neck, knees, hips, and even the temporomandibular joint. To help patients afflicted with this disease, we work with pediatric endocrinologists who understand that stabilizing the jaw will often stabilize the patient's posture and improve their airway. We are not "curing" this disorder, but simply providing palliative/supportive care and maintenance.

We also have relationships with pediatric psychologists, neurologists, sleep physicians, and pediatricians to help children suffering from depression, ADHD, and other disorders. For these children, we are able to provide solutions if part of their problem is a physical issue, such as a narrow airway. It is very common to find that airway issues are where patients' other issues stem from.

PERIODONTISTS

Helping a patient achieve normal function sometimes involves releasing a tied tongue, and we have a wonderful periodontist who is on our team for this purpose.

With this condition, the tongue is actually "tied" to the floor of the mouth by a short frenum, or that piece of flesh between the bottom of the tongue and the lower jaw. That attached tissue leaves the patient physically unable to get their tongue to rest in the roof of their mouth. When a person has a tied tongue, sometimes it will scrape across their lower front teeth when they try to stick out their tongue because it is attached in the middle in the front. Another presentation is that the sides of the tongue curl up and they end up with what looks like a heart-shaped tongue, because it's bound in the middle.

When the patient is an infant, we're able to release the tongue through an in-office procedure. It is quick and easy and requires no anesthetic. Having the mother breastfeed the child in a private room immediately following the procedure acts as myofunctional therapy. That post-release exercise and care are imperative and helps the procedure heal very quickly. The action of the tongue during breastfeeding, along with the mother conducting some simple exercise therapies, can help prevent scarring and keep the tongue from reattaching. Mothers really appreciate this when they are having difficulty nursing due to latching problems. By catching a tongue-tie problem early enough, we can get the child back on the road to proper development and health.

Tongue-tie is easier to fix when the problem is caught early on in childhood. But tongue-tie grows more complex as time goes on.

When patients with tongue-tie are older, they are referred out to a periodontist.

Myofunctional therapy can help a tongue-tie release procedure heal quicker and be more effective when it's performed on an adult. It also helps prevent reattachment after a procedure. For these reasons, and others, myofunctional exercises are performed before and after a tongue-tie release procedure. In our practice, myofunctional therapy is mandatory for these situations.

CHAPTER 8

The Muscles Are Boss (Myofunctional Therapy)

W hen Marla came in for a consult, she was diagnosed with having a very narrow nasal airway—the result of having a very narrow upper arch (since the roof of the palate is the floor of the nose). Instead of her tongue resting up against her palate, it was resting low and behind the lower teeth. The normal behavior of the facial muscles is for the cheek musculature to constantly put pressure at the sides of the mouth and on the teeth. Marla's cheeks exerted extra force due to poor muscle habits, which helped constrict her dental arches and drive the palate upward. If the tongue is not resting in the upper part of the mouth, the upper dental arch will become narrow—and that change can happen fairly rapidly. We needed to provide some orthodontic expansion to create enough room in Marla's palate for her tongue to fit.

In addition to orthodontic appliance therapy, Marla regularly performed myofunctional exercises as part of her treatment program, which helped expand her arch and open her nasal airway. The exercises helped balance out the function of her tongue, lips, and facial muscles. The result was a broad, healthy palate that allowed her tongue to posture nicely in the roof of her mouth.

Myofunctional therapy helps maximize and stabilize the treatments patients undergo and provides the best results. It consists of specialized exercises and behavior modification techniques designed to retrain the tongue, lips, jaw, and facial muscles. Myofunctional therapy can help correct and eliminate dysfunctional oral habits that may have repatterned facial muscles and negatively impacted the normal growth, development, and function of the face and jaws.

Through myofunctional therapy, patients relearn where the tongue should reside inside the mouth while at rest and how the tongue should function when drinking, chewing, and swallowing.

While there are a number of exercises under the myofunctional therapy umbrella, the actual exercises incorporated into any treatment are determined by patient needs—every patient doesn't use every exercise as part of their program. A thorough evaluation prior to therapy determines what is needed. This is a fluid situation and may be modified depending how the therapy is proceeding; adaptations and adjustments are made along the way.

Myofunctional Therapy for Lip Strength

Lip position and underlying muscle strength and tone are key to proper facial function. In the perfect circumstance, the lips should be touching together and the mouth closed most of the time, including when at rest or when swallowing. Lips should only be apart when eating, speaking, or smiling.

Myofunctional therapy can help strengthen lip muscles and retrain them to be in the proper position.

For instance, when a patient has an anterior open bite, the back teeth touch together and the front teeth do not. That happens because the tongue rests low inside the lower jaw or between the teeth. Without adequate lip muscle function and tone, a person's mouth may be open all the time, causing them to breathe through their mouth instead of their nose. If a patient has to work to get their lips together during the day, then their lips won't be together at night when they're asleep and their body is relaxed. Again, they'll breathe through their mouth once they are asleep, instead of using their nose.

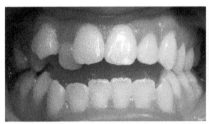
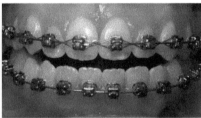

Before treatment   During treatment

If the lip muscles become flaccid from being apart too much, they actually need training to be strengthened so they can maintain their closed posture. In fact, lips sometimes appear shorter and less plump because the muscles don't have the normal tone—that happens especially with the upper lip. Performing the correct myofunctional exercises can change the muscle tone of the lip, effectively lengthening the muscle and making it easier to keep the lips together at rest.

Like Marla, patients may come in for a consultation, and after a comprehensive evaluation and diagnosis, the treatment recommendation is for orthodontic treatment to develop their arches. Even when that development structurally changes the arches, most patients still need myofunctional therapy to help them normalize the facial muscles and tongue posture for long-term success. By changing the structure and strengthening the muscles so that the lips more naturally close while at rest, the patient will ultimately be able to breathe better through their nose. Since breathing through the nose is a "use-it-or-lose-it" proposition, the airway will actually improve over time, as it's used more and more, following the structural and muscular changes. Of course, this is dependent upon the nose first becoming functional by creating a patent nasal airway for them.

Myofunctional Therapy in Kids

Sometimes, with children, we can already see that they have "left the highway," so to speak. Their facial growth is becoming abnormal, but it isn't beyond relatively straightforward help. We can still help them find the entrance ramp by instituting myofunctional therapy. Sometimes, myofunctional therapy can be a stand-alone treatment, especially with younger children.

The symptoms that myofunctional therapy can address in children (and in adults as well) include:

- mouth-breathing

- tongue thrust

- low tongue position

- forward head posture

- teeth clenching and grinding (bruxism)

- abnormal chewing and swallowing habits

- poor sleeping patterns

- thumb-sucking

- nail-biting

- open-mouth posture

Myofunctional therapy may also help reduce problems stemming from poor function of the facial muscles, including TMJ and sleep-breathing disorders. This treatment can eliminate symptoms arising from these dysfunctions, ranging from allergies to ADHD.

As discussed in Chapter 6, myofunctional exercises are an integral part of our treatment with the Myobrace appliances. The tongue is nature's palatal expander, and it especially effective when a child is still growing. Myofunctional therapy with Myobrace can help normalize the tongue posture to where it is positioned correctly in the mouth. When the mouth is closed, this position is on the palate, resting on the soft tissue behind the upper front teeth. That makes the upper jaw and the whole nasal maxillary complex grow wider and more forward, the way it's supposed to grow.

Often, intervening with myofunctional therapy and Myobrace early on gets kids "back on the right highway." Children whose facial structures may have them headed for a world of discomfort and low self-esteem can instead have lives with faces that are in balance and that grow to their full genetic potential. They look great. They function and sleep normally. The causes of crooked teeth are addressed early on, and they will usually not need braces. They are healthier and happier.

Myofunctional Therapy for Adults

Myofunctional therapy is also an essential part of the corrections for many adults.

Often, adult patients have aberrant functions that are simply adaptations the brain has figured out "just to make everything work." If, for instance, the tongue can't fit up in the palate where it allows for proper breathing and swallowing, then the brain figures out how to change the posture of the facial muscles and even the entire body to function to allow breathing to be as normal as possible. Often the adaptation leads to mouth breathing and aberrant swallow patterns.

To correct the problem, many adults need their neuromuscular pathways—those connections between the brain and the muscles—changed in order to begin to function normally and make all the structural corrections we are making stable. In adults, that can mean making corrections to the jaw that sometimes are beyond the ability of simple orthodontic techniques to achieve. There are some more extreme protocols that can achieve that kind of jaw correction, but many adults don't want to appear in public, even part time, wearing the appliances required to make that much correction. Some of these methods require wearing an appliance that is visible in front of the lips for twelve consecutive hours, every day. That is a big commitment that some adults have difficulty accepting.

With adults, treatment with Myobrace and myofunctional therapy doesn't involve the appliance itself significantly growing new bone. Following the Myobrace protocols, including the assigned exercises, will lead to the remodeling of bone. That remodeling occurs because the appliance promotes arch development and ideal function while it is being worn. The myofunctional exercises change the functional matrix, which then causes changes in structure. Melvin Moss supports the idea that "form follows function."[35] What that means for facial development is that the spaces inside the mouth and the functional requirements of those spaces dictate how the bone forms around the tongue and its movements, and the functional airway at the back of the mouth. Normalizing function from the old adaptive aberrant function requires the bones to be changed, and those changes promote continued bone remodeling toward the proper form. For example, let's say an adult finishes our orthodontic treatment at age forty-seven

---

35   ML Moss, "The functional matrix hypothesis revisited. 1. The role of mehanotransduc-
      tion," *Am J Orthod Dentofacial Orthop.* 112, no. 1 (July 1997): 8–11.

and is able to function closer to ideal than they had previously been able to. If they were x-rayed ten years later, their facial structure would have continued to remodel even more toward the ideal, because they had been functioning normally during that ten-year period of time. Time and function allows the bone to remodel to a more ideal form. That is the beauty of what we do: As we get people back on the path of normal function, their body and nature take over and continue the improvements.

Healing Tongue-Tie

As mentioned in the last chapter, myofunctional therapy will help in the healing process after tongue-tie surgery. Tongue-release surgery involves actually releasing or resecting the frenum, (that band of tissue holding the tongue to the floor of the mouth).

Achieving the best outcome for tongue-release in children and adults involves using myofunctional exercises before and after the surgery. Specific exercises must be done, depending on the location of the release and the tongue's function. The exercises before the procedure let the muscles know what they are supposed to do. This is sometimes difficult because the "tied" condition can prevent full function. The presurgery exercises also allow the patient to actively position their tongue which helps to provide better surgical access and a better ability to evaluate what must be released. The patient is able to hold their tongue up and out of the way. The exercises are also done after the procedure to help with healing and to maximize gains. The normal healing process can involve scar tissue formation and tissue shrinkage/retraction at the surgical site. Patients who don't do the exercises may lose a significant amount of the increases in ranges of motion that the surgeon created. More than half the intended correction may be lost by reattachment of the tie. Sometimes those reductions in mobility ranges can prevent normal function and lead to needing a repeat of the surgical procedure. The final result needs to allow the tongue to posture and move the way it's supposed to. There can also be lip ties that need to be released in some patients.

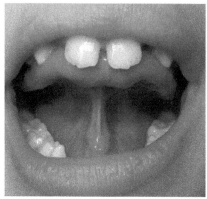 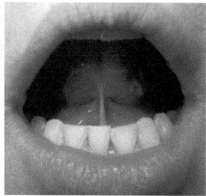

Child tongue tie   Adult tongue tie

In-Office Myofunctional Therapy

While some patients are referred out to a local periodontist who has a myofunctional therapist on staff, we are fortunate to also have an on-staff chiropractor who is certified as a myofunctional therapist. The periodontist we work with is very happy to utilize our myofunctional therapist.

She has been very helpful in "tweaking" her skills with regard to supporting his surgical procedures. She leads patients through the protocols and progressive exercises and helps track their progress. Having someone readily available to direct patient care helps them be more cooperative and more compliant. Patients also appreciate the convenience of being able to combine orthodontic and myofunctional therapy appointments. You can learn more about Dr. Kelly Wells by going to our website: drlipskis.com.

Myofunctional therapy is a critical treatment that most orthodontists don't offer patients, and that's one reason "traditional" orthodontic efforts often don't actually fix the problems patients have. We feel it is important that all of our orthodontic patients receive a full myofunctional evaluation eight weeks into their orthodontic treatment. Without myofunctional therapy and normalizing function, orthodontic treatment has been shown to be significantly less stable than it should be.

CHAPTER 9
Nutrition and Inflammation— The Connections

John, a dentist who practices in Florida, had attempted for more than a decade to treat himself for his TMJ pain and symptoms. He had successfully treated his own patients but couldn't seem to get the same protocols he was using to work for himself.

For twenty years, he had experienced considerable lower back pain, finally resorting to chiropractic and physical therapy visits twice or more each week just to "keep him functional." Since he hadn't been able to fix the source of his problems—his TMJ—the therapies for his back weren't offering any long-term relief. He finally decided that being a dentist and hunching over a dental chair with back pain was just part of life.

We met John about twenty years ago and had seen each other regularly at meetings and educational events. In 2015, he finally reached out to us for treatment. It was fun working with him—we both learned a lot. It took about an hour to work our way through all of his orthotics and various shoes to figure out that he really had a TMJ primary injury. He had been wearing foot orthotics for years "to help his back." Although he had never previously considered apnea as a part of his problems, Dr. Lynn investigated the issue, and John was diagnosed with mild OSA. She successfully provided treatment for John's TMJ and sleep apnea simultaneously.

John noticed immediate improvements from wearing his daytime orthotic and nighttime sleep appliance. Within two weeks, he was waking in the morning refreshed and his lower back pain had begun to subside.

Part of our discussion with him had also focused on his eating habits and the inflammation his food choices were causing. So he "got religion" by following an anti-inflammatory diet, which he followed faithfully for about three or four months. He was feeling great and we communicated regularly with him. Then he went on a "boys' trip," during which the group stopped at a burger joint. "What could it hurt?" John thought and joined in, "fudging a little." He learned a lot that night—his food choices affected his nasal airway so much that he tossed and turned all night. The next morning, he declared *never again*. That was several years ago and to this day he maintains his health by eating correctly. John is a great example of how much our personal choices affect how we feel.

A lot of patients who come to the practice don't even realize they have a breathing issue. They don't realize they're tired and cranky all the time. They only know they are in a lot of pain. If a patient who has had an obstructed airway their whole life is asked whether they can breathe well, often they will answer: "Yes, I breathe fine, I can breathe through my nose." But once their airway improves, then they understand the difference.

Often the reason for an obstruction is inflammation—that's

just one of the problems that inflammation causes. When the airway is inflamed, a cascade of other problems occurs. Ultimately, those problems culminate in chronic pain.

Inflammation can come from a variety of issues, but diet is one of the bigger factors. We also must consider allergies, environment, and habits.

Many physicians today are pointing to inflammation as one of the biggest enemies that they are waging battle against. As discussed in Chapter 2, our diets have been progressively getting worse over time because of the mistaken idea that eating fat was unhealthy. In truth, the problems have been caused by eating too much sugar, processed food, and unhealthy carbohydrates. When fat is taken out of the diet, it is too often substituted with sugar to make the food palatable. That has made society as a whole even fatter, less healthy, more inflammatory, and more susceptible to diseases than ever before.

TMJ Dysfunction and Inflammation

A malfunctioning TMJ is commonly a source of inflammation. It's like a little inflammation-producing machine. Every time you swallow, talk, or chew, the TMJ creates inflammation because the joint is not working correctly. Unfortunately, the inflammation doesn't stay put in that area. It travels through other parts of the body.

Inflammation is a bit of a double-edged sword. The body needs inflammation in the short term, to heal. Chronic inflammation, when an area is constantly inflamed, ultimately diminishes blood flow and compromises the nutrients going to that area. That results in tissue breakdown in that area over time. It causes the release of inflammatory factors that affect all the tissue in that area, enter the blood stream, and cause wide-reaching effects.

Just as chronic and acute pain are different (see Chapter 3), chronic and acute inflammation are not the same. If you bump your elbow, it swells up because that's part of the healing response to repairing injured tissues. That type of swelling is an inflammatory response that battles infection, for instance, from a cut or scrape. Acute inflammation is a good thing; it's the white blood cells in the body racing to the site of an injury to help with healing—that's what causes the swelling and inflammation.

Too much inflammation is a bad thing, however, which is why physicians will have you ice an injured site to keep the inflammation in check. When the inflammatory response becomes persistent or chronic, it leads to all kinds of issues. One way it can be detrimental to the body is because of its effect on pH level. Normally, we maintain an internal body pH at around a 7.3 to 7.4. Around the inflamed areas, that pH begins to drop and begins to become more acidic in the area. It can also lower pH in other areas of the body that have other sources of inflammation—that's when the problem becomes chronic and painful. Low pH can affect basic biochemical function that is designed to take place in the 7.3–7.4 range. Chronically, lower pH can even lead to bone breakdown in the affected area because the body breaks down bones to release calcium carbonate to alkalinize an area.

Let's use the TMJ as an example. Every time that injured joint moves (swallowing, talking, chewing), new inflammation is created. Over time, the effect of inflammation is the breakdown of the tissues surrounding the bones, or the bones themselves. Patients sometimes come in with a jaw joint that looks like it has worn away or been eaten away—the bone is actually being destroyed as a result of the chronic inflammatory state. So, when a patient asks, "Will it get worse if I do nothing?" our answer is an emphatic YES.

Add to that a diet loaded with carbohydrates and you're essentially throwing gasoline on a fire. While the source of the inflammation may be the TMJ, that inflammation can travel to other parts of the body from there, leading to chronic and even deadly diseases. When an injury increases inflammation somewhere in the body, it increases it everywhere, to some degree. The good news is that reducing the inflammation at the source—for example, the TMJ—generally reduces inflammation throughout the body.

> **-itis:** diseases ending in this suffix refer to inflammation of a certain body part, i.e. appendicitis, hepatitis, tendonitis, arthritis, etc.

This again, illustrates how everything in the body is connected. That's why some people begin feeling better right away with our treatment, because eliminating some of the demands/stress upon the body can help lower the demand/stress in other areas. The body has the ability to adapt. When stresses exceed that ability to adapt, a person feels like their body is falling apart, like it's breaking down. But what's really happening is that they're experiencing an overwhelming series of accumulated injuries and insults to the body. From a neurologic standpoint, we refer to this as "sensitization." Central sensitization can cause the brain to react illogically to stimuli, as with allodynia. Allodynia is a condition where the brain perceives a mild stimulus (like clothing touching your skin) as a much more severe stimulus, such as pain. If we can lighten some of that load and get that back into their adaptive range, then their symptoms will subside everywhere.

Addressing Inflammation

Technologies today make it possible to generate visual images of the inflammation in a person's body. Testing with magnetic resonance imaging (MRI) is the gold standard for revealing inflamed soft tissue. An MRI is not as effective at evaluating boney changes or "the big picture" as it is very focused imaging. Thermography is a photograph which shows areas that are warmer (warmer means inflammation). Our in-house cone beam computed tomography (CBCT) 3-D scanner creates images that can show the effects of inflammation on the air passages (swollen soft tissue), and we can create a virtual tour through the patient's airway. It can be an eye-opening experience for patients. We also can examine the TMJs, cervical spine, sinuses, etc.

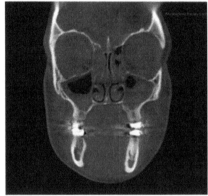 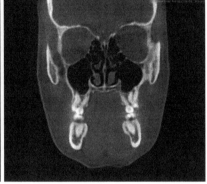

Blocked nasal airway and sinuses   Healthy nose and sinuses

Using i-CAT imaging software, we can reconstruct the anatomy of a patient's head and neck in 3-D. Regular CT scans only create individual slices of the airway. But with i-CAT, we can image the nasal airway from the tip of the nose. It is like "taking a stroll" through their airway. That allows us to see where the soft tissue is inflamed and blocking the nasal airway. We can also perform a volumetric analysis of the oropharyngeal airway.

In some patients, addressing the inflammation comes first. We do that through dietary suggestions, nasal sprays, orthotics, and other treatments or referrals. Some patients appear to eat healthy diets and have good overall health habits, but they still struggle to breathe because of food or environmental allergies. Oftentimes our orthodontic treatment can vastly change the patient's nasal airway and improve their tongue posture, giving them the ability to breathe much better. But if posttreatment i-CAT imaging reveals that mucosal tissue is still filling their now-enlarged nasal passages, then their food choices may actually be unhealthy for their particular body, or an environmental factor is creating challenges for them. Controlling the inflammation at that point requires further testing for food or environmental allergens, followed by dietary or other changes. We had one patient whose food allergy testing revealed that they are allergic to turmeric and flax seed—two foods that are considered extremely healthy!

The order of treatment depends on the patient. For instance, when Joey came in for an evaluation at age eleven, he had already been diagnosed with sleep apnea. An examination of his throat found tonsils and adenoids so enlarged that they were severely blocking his airway. It really was an emergency situation for him. The problem had already been noted and a sleep apnea diagnosis made a couple of years earlier by his pediatrician, who suggested at that time that he have his tonsils and adenoids removed. He never had the procedure, however, because his mother was anti-surgery. I also recommended surgical intervention to provide an immediate "fix." I was concerned with the serious short-term airway threat. Again, his mother declined surgery. Joey's only remaining option was to completely eliminate wheat, dairy, and sugar from his diet—a complete transformation to anti-inflammatory foods. His mother agreed to follow a strict diet for him, but at age eleven, it was doubtful he'd be entirely compliant.

Two weeks later, when Joey returned, the transformation was amazing! The size of his tonsils and adenoids had virtually normalized, his snoring was gone, and he no longer had apneic events—he no longer stopped breathing in his sleep, gasping for breath multiple times every hour. He was sleeping well and felt great. His results proved that he was onboard and compliant. What a wonderful change!

For Joey, following a strict, anti-inflammatory diet completely eliminated his symptoms. Somehow, his mother had managed to control his diet to the point that it literally saved his life. Most *adults* don't have that level of extreme restraint, even though diet can make a significant difference in their ability to breathe. It can be much more difficult for children.

Each case is different. Each person is different. When bone destruction is evident, as is often the case with TMJ problems, then appliance therapy is initially going to help more than dietary changes. If a nasal airway is structurally sound, yet blocked with inflammatory tissue, then steps are taken to begin reducing inflammation in the patient. That may include a referral to a nutritionist or an ENT/allergist.

In Joey's case, no other professional intervention was required. Some patients, however, put dietary compliance at the bottom of their list of priorities. While some patients with better diets don't have a lot of inflammation and benefit more from structural changes, others are so inflamed they can't breathe at all through their nose. Virtually every person has some room for improvement in their diet.

Foods That Cause Inflammation and Allergic Reaction

Patients are often surprised to learn some of the foods that can be inflammatory.

Grains. One of the most inflammatory categories of foods are grains. While some people can consume small amounts of wheat or other grains without any real inflammatory reaction, others are so sensitive that they get inflammation if even small amounts of grains have been used in the production of foods and certain vinegars, sauces, and liquors.

Gluten. Foods containing gluten can be some of the most inflammatory. Generally, gluten is part of a grain. Even though a person may not be diagnosed with celiac disease (an autoimmune disorder sometimes referred to as an "allergy" to gluten), a lot of people will react to gluten by experiencing increased inflammation. This would fall under the category of a sensitivity to gluten. "Gluten-free" eating has become popular because so many people who adopt it find that they feel better. Symptoms range from: fatigue/malaise, diarrhea, gas, constipation, achy joints, and brain fog. I often recommend that my patients read *Wheat Belly* by Dr. William Davis, or *Grain Brain* by Dr. David Perlmutter to get more detailed information about how foods can affect our health.

Dairy. Dairy products promote mucus production, which inflames and clogs the nasal passages. There are mixed reviews on whether people should consume dairy products and to what extent. I recommend an elimination diet to see how it affects you.

Processed carbohydrates. These include pasta, breads, cookies, candies, and other such foods. People often believe that whole wheat bread is better than white bread, but whole wheat bread is actually just as inflammatory because of the carbohydrate in wheat, known as amylopectin A. Similarly, people often think brown rice is a better choice than white rice because it provides more roughage, nutrients, and fiber. But for many people, the opposite is true because the husk of brown rice (like whole wheat) contains the proteins and allergens that can cause inflammation.

Alcohol (red wine). People who have sleep apnea are assured a bad night's sleep after drinking alcohol. Even though red wine from a health standpoint has some positive aspects to it, such as resveratrol, people with sleep apnea must get those positive aspects from other sources. Red wine actually targets the nasal membrane, causing swelling and limiting the opening for air flow. This inflammation can last six to eight hours, ruining a full night's sleep. Maybe we need to think about wine with lunch (just kidding)!

Acidic foods. Did you know that some bottled waters are almost as acidic as Coca Cola? That's a terrifying fact. Acidity causes inflammation. So, for some people, a diet that is higher in alkaline foods is the key to reducing inflammation. We provide our patients with handouts illustrating important facts like these.

Refined sugars. Sugar is everywhere. While fruit, for example, contains naturally occurring fructose, the fiber content partially offsets that negative feature. The less fiber in a fruit, the less healthy it is. The more fiber, the lower the glycemic index associated with that fruit, which is better. Fruit juices are also unhealthy. Drinking orange juice is not as good as eating an orange. You're going to get more sugar into your bloodstream faster drinking orange juice. That can affect your blood insulin levels and even lead to Type II diabetes.

The bottom line is that different diets work for different people because everyone processes food differently. You've probably heard the children's nursery rhyme that starts off "Jack Sprat could eat no fat; his wife could eat no lean"? That's entirely true. Some people need more fat to slow down the speed at which they process food, others thrive on eating very lean meats.

Any nutritional changes must be tailored to the individual because there is no one-size-fits-all solution when it comes to diet. That's why people get confused with fad diets—what works for one often doesn't work for another. It's really a journey of discovery that is difficult for most people to get onboard. When it comes to nutrition, we often refer patients to other resources. Some of these are local nutritionists, books, and journals.

Grandma used to say, "Eat your meat and vegetables, and if you're good, you'll get dessert." We should be eating what grandma said, which was a normal, balanced diet of real food, not processed foods. People who eat well can attest to that. It's tough to avoid the occasional bagel, bag of Doritos, or glass of red wine. But going off the wagon, so to speak, can lead to immediate inflammation. And for some, it can lead to a night of snoring or a longer-term bout of arthritis.

Most patients go to providers who don't address any of these issues, much less get help with the underlying origins of the problem. If the problem that started all the issues is not being addressed, how can any of the problems go away? That's what makes our practices different.

CHAPTER 10

What Sets Us Apart

A t the TMJ & Sleep Therapy Centre of Chicago and the Centre for Integrative Orthodontics, we take the time to help patients understand that everything in the body is connected. Then, we either address the issues affecting the patient or guide them to providers that can give them the help they need. As the "quarterback" for their care, we often help guide treatment priorities between ourselves and other providers, ensuring that the issues patients face are treated in the order that promotes the best and quickest healing.

Patients commonly comment on how much extra time and attention they receive from us. Our approach includes open communication with patients, and when needed, with other providers. That's the best way to begin eliminating chronic pain, airway issues, and the best path in improving a patient's quality of life.

Diagnosis Determines Treatment

We ask a lot of questions to help us make the connections we need to determine the proper diagnosis because that's what it all boils down to when treating patients—getting to the source of the problem.

Although treatment often involves some of the same or similar therapies used by other practitioners—an oral appliance, for instance—there is so much more involved in getting healthy through our protocols. And that starts with the diagnosis. It's not just the appliance that treats a TMJ problem, it's how it's used and the specific way it repositions a jaw that allows for a reduction in inflammation and the opening of an airway. The "same" appliance may not help at all, or can even make things worse, if it's not made to the doctor-determined, correct specifications for a particular patient's unique needs.

For instance, just as a splint on a broken bone holds it in place until it heals, the oral appliances we use are specially designed therapeutic orthopedic devices. These aren't just plastic mouth guards that protect the teeth from damage. They are orthotics individually designed and created to each patient's needs. They are designed to decompress the jaw joint, position the condyle as ideally as possible, and open the oropharyngeal airway. The patient is able to continue using their jaw while wearing the device and doing so helps reduce inflammation in the joint and promotes bone remodeling. We encourage normal function, rarely putting people on a "soft diet."

The amount of correction resulting from the device is determined from an in-depth evaluation and accurate diagnosis.

Comprehensive, Integrated Care

We have three very skilled practitioners who work together to provide the best care we possibly can. While we practice in one building, we're actually two separate practices offering comprehensive, integrated care in two very different environments.

The TMJ & Sleep Therapy Centre of Chicago is a very peaceful, tranquil environment that installs a sense of calm. That's because patients coming in for evaluation and Phase I treatment tend to be in a sympathetic, fight-or-flight state. They're already overstimulated when they walk through the door, so the goal from the minute they enter the practice is to help them begin feeling a sense of calm, support, and comfort. That's a crucial component to the start of their healing journey.

The Centre for Integrative Orthodontics is a more high-energy environment. Here, where integrative orthodontic and TMJ Phase II treatment occurs, patients tend to be more cheerful and upbeat when they walk through the door. They've recovered most of their health, so they're already in a better place before they embark on this part of their journey. And the treatment continues that trend—as their nasal airway improves, so does their ability to breathe. And that makes everything better. The Myobrace department which we also refer to as "The Kid's Centre" is designed specifically for kids from three to thirteen.

For instance, as treatment corrects deficiencies, such as in the upper lip, it actually improves the facial appearance for many patients. As their bone grows forward and leaves more room for the tongue, it opens the airway, opens the nasal passages, allows the patient to sleep better, and helps them appear more alert and more awake. Adults, especially, who have seen themselves aging for several years, suddenly find that they look and feel better and younger.

That's what happened to Sharon. She originally had a hard time committing to orthodontic treatment since she is a college professor and was concerned with her appearance. She also moved to Texas and now travels every one to three months for her orthodontic treatment. But on one such visit, she actually commented, "I wouldn't mind wearing these braces for a long time because I feel so great!" Still, she is looking forward to her much-improved life when her treatment wraps up, which should be completed within the next few months.

Since today's technologies allow for less pain with treatment, patients don't dread a visit to the practice. Again, the Damon System uses only 20 percent of the force of traditional braces, and is non-inflammatory, so adjustments are much more comfortable. The cold laser we use helps reduce or eliminate any inflammatory response.

For patients who are experiencing an inflammatory flare-up, the Centre also has a private room available. That's sometimes needed for patients whose journey is longer and/or a little more complicated.

The Patient Experience

Our patients are special people. They become part of the family. Our mantra is "How can we help?"

Rewards are also part of the program at the center. We strive to make it a positive experience. For example, children may receive a T-shirt for doing their myofunctional exercises, and they can earn points for good oral hygiene, or for wearing their Orthodontic Centre's T-shirt on appointment days. Those points can be redeemed for literally thousands of items available online.

A very thorough exam is essential to the comprehensive protocol at our practices. We spend time talking with each new patient to learn more about their lifestyle, sleep habits, medical history, and so forth.

TMJ and orthodontic patients are evaluated in private rooms, with parents accompanying young patients. Adult patients are also encouraged to bring a family member or friend with them. Another set of ears is always beneficial to help listen and potentially help the patient better understand our protocol.

That can be very helpful, especially in the first visit, because our practice is very different. While a patient may come in believing they have one issue that needs to be addressed—crooked teeth, for example— what we're going to talk about is what's causing their problem. We believe that crooked teeth are a symptom of a bigger problem. That is different than most dental practices, where the evaluation looks only at the complaint and makes the diagnosis based upon that.

In our practice, the evaluation may lead to a diagnosis that the teeth are crooked because of an airway obstruction, TMJ, myofunctional disorder, or an injury somewhere else in their body that's causing them to clench. Crooked teeth are just a symptom of a problem that has caused their body to change. Without getting to the origin of the problem, the issue is not truly corrected and any treatment ultimately will not be stable.

In fact, treatments that don't target the source may actually worsen existing problems, leaving the patient feeling and even looking worse than before they sought treatment. Our treatments make the patient skeletally more symmetrical, more stable, and more ideal. When the facial structure is more ideal, then the patient is able to function better.

After talking with patients about their history, their lifestyle, and their habits, they are then put through a comprehensive set of tests to get an accurate diagnosis. While adults can often more accurately articulate their symptoms, children aren't always as accurate in their descriptions. Testing for them is best done using technology but may also be as simple as asking them to walk with their mouth closed to see how many steps they can go through just breathing through their nose (for many, it's only a few steps).

Here are some of the tests and technologies we use to arrive at an accurate diagnosis:

Photographs. Most orthodontists take eight photographs of a patient's face. We take twenty photographs of the face and full body. That provides us information such as whether a patient has forward head posture and other postural compensations. When we see that, we want to know why. Looking for answers to those kinds of questions is what helps our patients get healthier.

Muscle palpation. This is a thorough physical exam of the head and neck that checks different muscles. Light pressure is applied to muscles to test for sensitivity, which helps us diagram what muscles may be responsible for aberrant function. Patients and their companions are often surprised at how a light pressure can cause pain.

Intraoral exam. This is a visual exam to ensure that nothing in the mouth will negatively impact the treatment, or will be negatively impacted by treatment. The visual exam looks for crowded or loose teeth, the number of teeth intact and missing, excessive wear on the teeth, tongue-ties, tongue size and function, scalloped tongue, the size and condition of the airway, or keratinization that would indicate chewing on the cheek, and so on.

Breathing issues. We perform tests to check the patient's breathing and may even refer them with an order for a home sleep study as a screening test. All sleep tests are reviewed by a certified sleep physician who then provides the diagnosis.

Posture. We evaluate posture passively (photographs) and actively (walking) so we can get "clues" as to how the person is adapting to their condition.

Motor nerve reflex testing. This is a system of neurologic reflex tests to locate physical injuries to certain parts of the body that are causing a neurologic response. Motor nerve reflex testing helps us determine if the patient has a structural issue and whether they are in a sympathetic state. It also helps us identify the origin of a problem when a patient comes in with a list of complaints. This helps us determine an accurate diagnosis and allows us to correctly treat people who actually have TMJ problems, not just TMJ symptoms related to a problem in another body part.

Joint vibration analysis (JVA). This is a computerized test. Small sensors are placed over the patient's jaw joint to record vibration in the joint as the patient opens and closes their mouth. The computer does an analysis based on the wavelength frequency and pattern of the vibration. This technology has been proven to be an accurate predictor of the condition of the joint. The JVA helps verify the findings of the physical and visual examinations.

Cone beam computed tomography (CBCT). CBCT produces a 3-D scan of the head, neck, and airway to help improve the accuracy of the diagnosis. During an imaging session, the scanner rotates around the patient's head to produce thousands of "slices" of images. The software then reconstructs the images to create three-dimensional images that make it easy for patients (and parents), and us as providers, to see volume in the airway and skeletal discrepancies. The software also includes a color-coded scale of the measure of the airway. This particular imaging machine is incredibly low in radiation.

Pharyngometer. This is a sonar test that checks the volume of the throat. The patient breathes through the machine, then they perform exercises designed to induce collapse of the airway. The sleep appliance is then inserted and the exercises are repeated to determine if the appliance can lessen the collapsibility. Anytime the collapsibility is lessened, the patient's airway is maintained better. The pharyngometer helps provide objective data to a sleep physician when making adjustments to a sleep appliance.

Patients on the Team

While we have a team of professionals in our offices, it's also crucial for the patient to, in essence, join the team. Peter, for example, was a patient who understood our protocols and achieved great success.

Thank you for the alternative treatment for my condition of sleep apnea. I had been attempting to use a CPAP machine without success. I found the full face mask to be very claustrophobic as well as the tubing to be very restrictive. Neither promoted restful sleep. As such I did not use the CPAP machine and my sleep apnea was not treated.

Your office completed a comprehensive assessment for treating my sleep apnea and prescribed a dental appliance. The appliance has been LIFE CHANGING and has exceeded my expectations. I am sleeping soundly through the night and waking well rested and refreshed. Additionally, I have appreciated your follow-up concerning the dental appliance. TMJ & Sleep Therapy Centre has set the gold standard for medical treatment. —**Peter**

The type of treatments we offer are not therapies we *do to patients*, they are treatments we use when *working with patients* to make them healthier. We expect people to become active in becoming healthier. That's what makes our program most effective, when a patient buys into the protocol and understands their role in returning to health.

CONCLUSION

Too often, patients want a quick-fix for their problems. They want to be able to take a pill to make their pains and ailments go away. In today's changing health care landscape, physicians are facing overwhelming financial and insurance pressures on top of the pressure from patients who just want the quick-fix. When a patient comes in, it's easier and quicker just to go straight to the area of their complaint. A patient claiming "my face hurts" may lead to little more than a prescription for a pain reliever.

But that's not the way to resolve the problem. The only way to truly resolve a body that's in a sympathetic state is to figure out and address the origin of the problem. In most health care situations, that's not done. The treatment ends up being a symptom-chasing approach. That may provide relief of some of the patient's symptoms, but it doesn't make their problem go away. In fact, some of these issues may only be masked, while the problem continues to cause further breakdown. By getting to the origin of the problem and addressing it, the symptoms are relieved and the patient actually gets healthier.

At the TMJ & Sleep Therapy Centre of Chicago and the Centre for Integrative Orthodontics, we don't chase symptoms. We look for the cause and then address it effectively.

Again, acute pain and acute injuries are obvious, so treatment and healing is a more direct process. Chronic pain is complex. It's usually a matter of dealing with multiple problems—some longstanding, some not—but many of which don't necessarily stem from an obvious source. In fact, when someone is in a sympathetic state, the origin of a structural problem is the most protected site, so that's the least likely place for the patient to have symptoms. Yet that protected site is the first place that needs to be addressed.

Chronic pain is not something that can be cured with a magic wand—or a magic pill. Even though we can create the environment for healing and can change the structures as needed to help patients feel better, it takes participation by the patient to return to wellness. Sometimes that means "managing" the issue, like we do with our patients that have chronic medical conditions like Ehlers-Danlos syndrome or surgically altered patients.

If you are suffering from chronic pain, we can help. But we need you to also take on the responsibility for your health. You are a key player on your wellness team. While we can improve your situation, you make the decision of just how well you want to be.

If you're tired of chronic pain and if you're tired of sleepless nights, join us in the journey to return to health. We can help you get your life back.

ABOUT THE AUTHORS

D rs. Edmund and Lynn Lipskis began a "thirty plus years" long "mini-crusade" as an effort to improve their lives personally. This crusade has expanded to inform the public of what they have learned in an effort to improve many more lives.

As a chronic pain sufferer, Dr. Lynn Lipskis was determined to find answers and embarked on a thirty-year journey with over five thousand hours of post-graduate, continuing education in the areas of facial development, orthodontics, facial orthopedics, craniofacial pain, and sleep medicine. She has studied TMJ and sleep apnea solutions extensively with Dr. John Witzig, Dr. Harold Gelb, Dr. Derek Mahony and Dr. Steven Olmos, and has studied physical therapy techniques with Dr. Mariano Rocobado and cranial osteopathy with Dr. Viola Frymann. She is a fellow of the American Academy of Craniofacial Pain. Dr. Lynn has also completed the requirements for and is board-certified with The American Board of Craniofacial Pain, has been board-certified with the American Board of Dental Sleep Medicine, and has a board-certified diplomate status in sleep dentistry with American Board of Craniofacial Pain Sleep Medicine. This triple board-certification is not common—there's maybe a total of two hundred individuals in the United States. Her interest and expertise in caring for children was enhanced while teaching at the Loyola University School of Dentistry in the Department of Pediatric Dentistry 1982 until 1993.

Dr. Edmund Lipskis has over five thousand hours of postgraduate education in the fields of orthodontics, dentofacial orthopedics, TMJ dysfunction, sleep-related breathing disorders, and chronic pain therapies. He travels worldwide to study with some of the leaders in these fields, including Drs. John Witzig, Derek Mahony, John and Michael Mew, Mariano Rocabado, and Steven Olmos. His training has helped him become very aware of the "need to breathe" and how he can positively impact his patients' lives. He is a board-certified diplomate of the American Board of Craniofacial Pain, a board-certified diplomate of the American Board of Craniofacial Dental Sleep Medicine, and a board-certified diplomate of The International Association of Orthodontics. This triple board-certification is very rare, with less than fifty others having it worldwide. He also is a Fellow of the American Academy of Craniofacial Pain, a Fellow of the International Association of Orthodontics, and a Fellow of the American Academy of Functional Orthodontics. In 2016, Dr. Ed was awarded the Haden Stack Award (the Heismann equivalent in the chronic pain therapy world).

Drs. Edmund and Lynn Lipskis host an annual course for doctors on Airway Focused/Integrative Orthodontic Treatment for TMD/Airway Focused Orthodontics, featuring a hands-on course with patients in their office. Dr. Lynn has also given presentations on "cold" laser therapy, sleep apnea, ADHD, and TMD to dental societies locally and nationally. Dr. Ed regularly lectures in the United States and internationally on Airway Driven Orthodontics and Phase II treatment via orthodontics for chronic pain individuals.

Their practice mission statement is "to make a profound positive impact on people's lives," and they always strive to make a difference. Annually, they participate in Children's Dental Health Month, Freedom Day for veteran's and Dentists with a Heart.

They are active in their community, and in 2017, they organized a dental mission trip to Belize with their staff. "Our staff was awesome at organizing everything pre-mission and the epitome of joyful workers during the long, hot days. We could not have done it without them."

OUR SERVICES

f you or someone you know suffers from any of the conditions below or discussed in this book, it's time to give us a call at the TMJ and Sleep Therapy Centre of Chicago and the Centre for Integrative Orthodontics.

- unexplained jaw pain or headache upon waking

- snoring (especially in children)

- waking suddenly at night, gasping for air

- grinding teeth at night

- bedwetting

- unresolved headaches, neck pain, back pain.

- malocclusion

- ADHD in children

- crooked teeth

There are alternatives to surgery to help you eliminate chronic pain, reduce/eliminate snoring and get a great night's sleep. With a comprehensive evaluation, we can make an accurate diagnosis and determine therapies that may include:

- a removable oral orthotic to three-dimensionally reposition the jaw to help reduce muscle fatigue and pain

- appliances to relieve snoring not caused by sleep apnea

- oral appliance therapy for obstructive sleep apnea

For patients who need additional therapy to make a corrected jaw position permanent, we also offer treatment that corrects facial asymmetries, functional issues like diminished airways and poor breathing, and structural/potentially painful issues of the face, including TMJ. These treatments include orthodontics, a removable bite restorer, crown and bridge restorations, and specialty dentures.

We achieve beautiful smiles with beautifully balanced faces, and we help people eliminate chronic pain, breathing disorders, and disrupted sleep, leading to healthier lives.

REACH OUT TO US AT:

TMJ and Sleep Therapy Centre of Chicago, 630-762-8700
The Centre For Integrative Orthodontics, 630-377-5600
www.drlipskis.com